T0215297

THE HEALTHY ANCESTOR

Advances in Critical Medical Anthropology
Series Editors: Merrill Singer and Pamela Erickson

This book series significantly advances our understanding of the complex and rapidly changing landscape of health, disease, and treatment around the world with original and innovative books in the spirit of Critical Medical Anthropology that exemplify and extend its theoretical and empirical dimensions. Books in the series address topics across the broad range of subjects addressed by medical anthropologists and other scholars and practitioners working at the intersections of social science and medicine.

Volume 1
Global Warming and the Political Ecology of Health: Emerging Crises and Systemic Solutions, Hans Baer and Merrill Singer

Volume 2
The Healthy Ancestor: Embodied Inequality and the Revitalization of Native Hawaiian Health, Juliet McMullin

THE HEALTHY ANCESTOR

Embodied Inequality and the Revitalization of
Native Hawaiian Health

Juliet McMullin

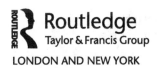

Routledge
Taylor & Francis Group

LONDON AND NEW YORK

First published 2010 by Left Coast Press, Inc.

Published 2016 by Routledge
2 Park Square, Milton Park, Abingdon, Oxon OX14 4RN
52 Vanderbilt Avenue, New York, NY 10017

Library of Congress Cataloging-in-Publication Data

McMullin, Juliet Marie.
  The healthy ancestor : embodied inequality and the revitalization of native hawaiian health / Juliet McMullin.
      p. cm.—(Advances in critical medical anthropology)
  Includes bibliographical references and index.
  ISBN 978-1-59874-499-6 (hardcover : alk. paper)
  ISBN 978-1-59874-500-9 (paperback : alk. paper)
  1. Medical anthropology—Hawaii. 2. Public health—Hawaii.
  3. Traditional medicine—Hawaii. 4. Hawaiians—Health and hygiene.
  5. Hawaiians—Medical care. 6. Hawaiians—Ethnic identity.
  7. Body, Human—Social aspects—Hawaii. I. Title.
  GN296.5.U6M35 2009
  306.4'6109969—dc22
  2009028844

Cover design by Piper Wallis.
Cover illustration "The Kalo" by Cameron Chun, pthaloblue.com

ISBN 13: 978-1-59874-500-9 (pbk)
ISBN 13: 978-1-59874-499-6 (hbk)

CONTENTS

PREFACE

When I arrived in Hawai'i in the mid-1990s to begin fieldwork, my original intent was to understand Native Hawaiian knowledge of cancer and specifically of breast cancer risks. At the time, Native Hawaiian women had some of the highest rates of breast cancer in the United States. The proposed work would be an extension of my work on cancer disparities among Latinas and, on a personal note, it would give me an opportunity to learn about my family who were from the islands. As I began talking with Native Hawaiian women and men I found that many were willing to share their stories of loved ones who had experienced and then passed away from cancer. What was of more interest to the people I spoke with, and the friends I made along the way, was their overall view of Hawaiian health. They were interested in how health was impacted by their lack of sovereignty and access to land and traditional healthy foods. This book is an effort to describe what Native Hawaiians told me about their health and the politics of health. It is my analysis of how Native Hawaiians describe the former and the continuing unraveling of their physical and cultural health by those who promote social structures that value dismembering social relationships and promote individual responsibility as the sole course of action. More importantly, it is a description of how on-island and off-island Native Hawaiians remember their ancestors through meanings of health and practices that reintegrate relationships with the 'āina and with each other. The practices associated with health and remembering are political statements against the inequities Native Hawaiians have suffered as well as a charter for their own views on how to be healthy and overcome cultural, political, and health inequalities.

There are two issues on language that should be clarified. The first is the use of the term *Native Hawaiian* as an ethnic identifier. There have been numerous terms used for this group: *Hawaiian, native Hawaiian, Native Hawaiian, Kanaka Maoli,* and *Kanaka Oiwi*. Silva (2004) and Kauanui (2008) have shown the historical and political use of these terms. For instance, *native Hawaiian* is used by the Federal Government to describe individuals who have a blood quantum of at least 50 percent Hawaiian ancestry to pre-contact Hawaiians (Hawaiians who lived on the islands prior to Captain Cook's arrival in 1778) (Kauanui 2008). In contrast, *Native Hawaiian* is used to signify any blood relationship to pre-contact Hawaiians. More recently, members of Hawaiian sovereignty and revitalization movements have used *Kanaka Maoli*, meaning *real people* to identify Native Hawaiians (e.g., Kame'eleihiwa 1992; Blaisdell 1993; Trask 1993; Gomes 1994). I have used all the terms to signify any individual with ancestry that traces back to pre-contact Hawaiians. The second note on language is the use of Hawaiian words. Following the lead of Native Hawaiian scholars (Silva 2004; Kauanui 2008), Hawaiian words are not italicized and definitions are provided at the first use of a word.

I am forever grateful to all the acquaintances, friends, mentors, and colleagues who provided endless encouragement in getting this book to publication. First and foremost are the people who generously shared their time and knowledge with me. I hope my understanding of your mānao is worthy of your care for me. Among those individuals is Carolyn Kuali'i who prompted me to begin this work and guided me throughout the process. To Clarence Kahana and Dorothy Kauahi who so generously opened their home to my daughter and me, we will always remember you as family. To Virginia and Angie who assisted with some of the interviews. Mahalo to, Kamuela Senior Center, Nā Mamo, Hui No Ka Ola Pono and Ka'anapali Hotel who were supportive of this effort. And to Cameron Chun whose artwork captured so many of the ideas I have tried to convey and who graciously allowed me to use *The Kalo* for the book cover. To my academic mentors Leo Chavez, Mike Burton, Art Rubel, Karen Leonard, and Carol Browner: thank you for reading numerous drafts as data was being collected and ideas were in their infancy. The Department of Social Relations at University of California, Irvine provided summer funding. My colleagues at the University of California, Riverside have been immensely supportive in the final effort to complete the manuscript. In particular, Tom Patterson for his gentle yet persistent questioning and encouragement during the different stages of theorizing and editing; Chikako Takeshita, Jennifer Heung, Sally Ness, Christina Schwenkel, and Amalia Cabezas were a sounding board for many thoughts about place and identity. To my haumana, Laurette McGuire, Lisa Garibaldi, and Amy Dao who read, critiqued, and assisted with obtaining images; you make teaching and learning so much fun. Merrill Singer and Pamela Erikson, editors of the Advances in Critical Medical Anthropology series at Left Coast Press, thank you for helping frame the book in a literature that finally made me let go; your questions and insights have been invaluable. Jennifer Collier, I am grateful for your encouragement, patience, and help through the whole publishing process.

For Mark and Sheila, the two of you have been my greatest supporters over the years. Sheila, who from the time we stepped off the plane in Hawai'i to this very moment, is sitting by my side, listening, encouraging, laughing. How did I end up with such an amazing child? Mark, for your undying support for all of my projects. I can't tell you what a privilege it's been to have you in my life. "Me he lau no ke Ko'olau ke aloha" ~ 'Ōlelo nóeau (Pukui 1983:234).

INTRODUCTION

When a Hawaiian says "Hawaiian culture," you gotta understand that he puts his culture with the land. The land is part of his genealogy...it's what makes you know. Maybe if people were to look at it, this association with nature and the land and everything in the sea and that it's yours and that you know you're a part of it. It's a special kind of healing that remains.

—Interview with Kalani

Once touted as the healthiest state in the nation, Hawai'i looms in the minds of Americans as a tropical paradise, a land of leisure and relaxation, a mentally and physically healthy place. The fact that Hawai'i was one of the only states to offer universal health coverage bolstered this perception. And yet, from the early encounters with Europeans and Americans to the present, colonists, missionaries, and state, federal, and local organizations have been documenting the increasingly poor health status of the indigenous population. Today, Native Hawaiians have a lower life expectancy; higher mortality rates for heart disease and cancer;[1] and higher age-adjusted morbidity rates for other chronic diseases such as diabetes, hypertension, and asthma than any other ethnic group in the state (Johnson, Oyama, and Marchand 1998; Office of Hawaiian Affairs 2006).[2] Attention to Native Hawaiian health or lack thereof has been further accentuated by the 100-year observance of the overthrow of the Hawaiian Monarchy in 1893. The stark contrast between claims of being one of the healthiest states in the Union (United Health Foundation 2004) and the impoverishment and misery of the indigenous population raises the following questions: For whom is this state healthy? What historical and social processes give rise to representations of individuals and groups as unhealthy? And, indeed, what do we even mean when we proclaim that a person or a group is or is not healthy?

Morbidity and mortality statistics are evidence enough that Native Hawaiians carry a greater burden of disease than other populations in the state. Often,

11

however, these statistics serve conflicted social purposes in that they can highlight economic and health inequalities, suggesting the need for structural changes to improve health and social well-being, as well as categorize individuals into groups in order to fault their beliefs and behaviors as problematic and as the primary sources of their health and social suffering (Foucault 1988; Crawford 1994). In their latter role, one performed within dominant ideologies in society—statistics as a tool for categorizing populations—statistics can be applied so as to help obscure alternative discourses of health and how to best achieve health. In the specific case of Hawai'i, understandings of health are central to Native Hawaiians' struggle for the restoration of their land, identity, and sovereignty.

One evening early in my fieldwork, the symbolic role of poi, the food made from the kalo or taro root, clarified an alternative discourse of health for me. For Melelani, dinner provided an opportunity to care for her family and friends and to show me the healthy foods Hawaiians eat. However, obtaining the cornerstone of the meal, poi, was problematic. A good portion of the day was spent sending friends to multiple stores to look for poi. During the mid-1990s, it was not unusual to see long lines of people waiting eagerly for the poi shipment at the grocery store. By mid-afternoon poi was scarce because most stores were already sold out. We scoured the shelves of three different stores before, finally, we were able purchase poi for our meal.

That evening, along with the poi, Melelani prepared chicken laulau (chicken that is first wrapped in taro leaves and then wrapped and baked in ti leaves), and lomi-lomi salmon (a tomato, onion, and salmon mix), which she said was not traditional Hawaiian food but that many people enjoyed and was very healthy. When the time came to prepare the poi, Melelani carefully cleaned a large bowl. She poured and then squeezed every remnant of poi out of its 16-ounce plastic bag. Melelani said that you had to be careful to respect the poi and not let any of it drip around the sides of the bowl. She then described what she watches for when other people eat poi. People who do not twirl the poi properly after picking it up with their fingers or a spoon and allow the poi to spill back into the bowl do not respect their ancestors, their family, or the land. She explained that kalo, the plant from which poi is made, is considered an elder sibling. You must respect your elders and the land that fed your ancestors so that it will continue to take care of and feed you. You must mālama 'aina (care for the land).

Kalo is a key symbol for many Hawaiians. Throughout my research I found that kalo encapsulates notions of identity, of the relationship Native Hawaiians feel toward each other and the land. Kalo is also a symbol of the foundation of indigenous health and survival. The reverence Melelani gave to poi (kalo) at our meal together exemplified many points that ultimately became meaningful during my research in Hawai'i. The ways in which Hawaiians categorized some foods as "Hawaiian" and "healthy" was not only an issue of physical health but also as served as a symbolic statement on the value of caring for family and ancestors, and the importance of the land, which in turn nourishes kalo. These three—land, kalo, and people—form an interlocked set, physically and spiritually, each caring for the others. The difficulty of finding poi also underscored how hard it can be for Native Hawaiians to get the very foods they define as essential to their health and identity. Dinner with Melelani opened a door for me into the important roles of food and land in how Native Hawaiians imagine their world, their health, their relationships, and their attempts to maintain and revitalize cultural ideals and heritage.

This book examines how concepts of "health" become meaningful and embodied aspects of cultural identity among Native Hawaiians. I view health as a continual process that is intimately tied to the larger historical and contemporary political economy and cultural knowledges that interact, producing and co-producing meaning. I examine the importance of the relationship between land and Hawaiian history, and the central role each of these play in giving meaning to an alternative model of Hawaiian health among Native Hawaiians living in Hawai'i (on-islanders). I then trace discourses of health, and their associations with land and history among Native Hawaiians living in Southern California (off-islanders). On-islanders and off-islanders both strive to maintain a Native Hawaiian culture and identity, but important shifts occur in their access to and definition of health, and the relative importance of health as a marker of "Hawaiianness." As suggested in Kalani's quote at the beginning of this chapter, health has been historically linked to relationships with land, foods, and family (past and present). Because these relationships may be less available in off-island locales, questioning the meaning of health focuses attention on current debates about transnational identities while simultaneously raising issues related to local political economies of health.

The question of how off-islanders can mālama 'āina (care for the land) when they do not live on the land of their ancestors is a question on the minds of some as highlighted in the lyrics of untitled track on *Call it What you Like . . .* by Mark Keali'i Ho'omalu (2003). His response to this question links land, body, and health for off-islanders who, like their counterparts in Hawai'i, do not always have access to the 'āina (land). By imagining Native Hawaiian bodies as the carriers of the 'āina caring for your body becomes the practical way to mālama 'āina. Through genealogy of people and land Ho'omalu maintains off-islanders' heritage as Kanaka 'Ōiwi (people of the bone) and yet, his response also draws on the science of DNA, which can be cited in debates over blood quantum and dispossession of Hawaiians from the 'āina, to create a genealogical relationship. As a result, a link between science and health is created that simultaneously integrates and fractures health and land associations by defining Hawaiian identity beyond the geographical space of Hawai'i through a reliance on biomedical technologies. The technologies used to define "Hawaiianness" and acknowledgment of caring for the land through the body are central to larger political debates on sovereignty, access to land, and cultural identity.

The processes that create the tension between health, land, and identity for on- and off-islanders are of primary concern for this research. These processes are clarified by examining the importance of a historical and cultural memory in the revitalization of an intertwined model of health and cultural identity, by exploring how each group (in Hawai'i and California) varies in its definitions of health and fluidity of identity, and by assessing the significance that each group attributes to health as part of daily life. Viewing health as part of daily life illuminates the co-production and contestation of the hegemony of biomedicine, the processes of medicalization, and the complex relationship between health and cultural identity. By examining an alternative model of health, and, in effect, an indigenous counter-hegemonic discourse, I am, unavoidably, offering up a critique of biomedical definitions and contemporary capitalism, or at least the ways in which capitalism leads to the commodification of health and body and characterizes gaping health inequalities as part of what is presumed to be a natural state of social relationships. In other words, within biomedicine and within capitalist social formations generally, health inequalities are often characterized as an outcome of individuals' essential natures rather than an issue of structurally imposed unequal access to resources and spaces that facilitate health. By examining other views, indigenous ones in the conflicted terrain of Hawai'i, I show how contemporary capitalism works to produce and naturalize inequity.

Health and Inequality: A Critical Medical Anthropology Approach

Work in critical medical anthropology (CMA) informs much of the present argument. Inasmuch as it is profoundly important for Native Hawaiians to remember and practice the forms of knowledge that they believe to be necessary and practical for the contemporary era, a CMA approach moves toward the integration of historical and political economic perspectives with cultural knowledge of health and illness (Morsy 1996; Baer, Singer, and Susser 2003). Combining a CMA approach with the revitalization of Native Hawaiian identities delineates power and resistance as well as the co-production of meanings of health within medical and identity processes. Following Nguyen and Peschard's 2003 argument that while statistics may make visible points where inequality occurs, in order to truly understand inequality in societies we must understand "how local actors understand, enact, and respond to inequalities and, as a result, how these translate into embodied effects (455)." For this work, the embodiment of inequality registers at both the representational level of national and cultural identities and at the individual level of health experiences and meanings of health.

Native Hawaiians' circumstances in Hawai'i underscore the importance of questions of health as well as the historical inequities that produced current struggles (see Chapter 1 for more historical information). For example, in 1962 the Lili'uokalani Trust Advisory Board published a report stating that Native Hawaiians were overrepresented in many of the categories of "social problems," which included low educational and economic attainment, high numbers of "illegitimate" children, and poor health status when compared to other ethnic groups in the state. This report prompted a number of studies that examined the daily lives of Native Hawaiians, focusing on beliefs and behaviors that improved or contributed to poor health and lower socioeconomic status.[3] Later studies continued to show startling rates of heart disease, cancer, diabetes, and accidents for Native Hawaiians (Alu Like 1985; Office Technology Assessment 1987; Wegner 1989). During the 1990s, Native Hawaiians had the lowest life expectancy, higher mortality rates for heart disease and cancer, and higher age-adjusted morbidity rates for other chronic diseases such as diabetes, hypertension, and asthma (Johnson, Oyama, and Marchand 1998). This trend has persisted throughout the present decade (Office of Hawaiian Affairs 2006). These studies are a double-edged sword. They are helpful because they provide valuable information about inequality and suffering in Native communities. If we take these studies and statistics at face value, however, they suggest that more should be done to bring multiple facets of Native Hawaiians' social life under the medical gaze. This process of medicalization ignores the historical and structural power relations that produced existing social and health inequalities (Waitzkin 1983; Martin 1992; Baer, Singer, and Susser 2003).

The process of medicalization also permits what Farmer (1999) calls the "mistaking of inequality for cultural difference." In the same way that medicalization shifts the blame from social structure to individual, focusing on cultural beliefs and practices as the source of poor health outcomes obscures the role of the political economy in health inequalities. For example, King (1987) has argued that the focus on "unhealthy" Hawaiians has contributed to the problem of adequately representing Native Hawaiians' health status. She notes that an unintended consequence is the prevailing view that Native Hawaiians are inherently or "naturally" unhealthy. The historical and social relations that gave rise to high rates of disease are rarely included in these discussions. Yet, mortality statistics and reports of "unhealthy" behaviors are used to represent Native Hawaiians as having a "lack of self-control" and of their "failure to progress." These negative characterizations are reminiscent of the role of biomedicine in the colonizing process across the Pacific.[4] As described by Anderson (2006), American techniques of health and hygiene were employed in the Philippines in the 1920s and 1930s as part of the civilizing process for Filipinos. Like Native Hawaiians, Filipinos were characterized by the Americans as "filthy" and "as children" in need of training (2006:107). The characterizations of these groups depend on using definitions of health to create a distinction, a difference between who is and is not civilized. Thus, "race" and biology become a "natural" foundation for the taking of resources and the exercise of political power. As such, these representations mistake inequality for cultural difference by using culture to obscure inequalities in access to health care as well as alternative definitions and practices of health.

The associations between colonialism, Native Hawaiian health statistics, and representations of cultural "failings" give us insight into the exercise of power through discourses of knowledge (Foucault 1979) and suggest a pattern of structural violence. Exposing relationships of structure and power illuminates the ways in which the social structure (including cultural, institutional, political, and economic ideologies and practices) constrain Native Hawaiian agency, hindering individuals and groups from acquiring healthy foods and accessing healthy environments (Farmer 1999, 2003). As discussed in Chapter 1, some of the structural factors that facilitate the violence in Hawai'i include the political subordination of Hawaiian medical knowledge and practices and the alienation of Hawaiians from their land, both of which created much of the poverty that many Natives currently experience. Structural violence is achieved "by allowing affliction to be related to prevailing ideologies that inform policy, configurations of social violence, the way misfortune is conceptualized and managed, and how meaning systems influence how individuals interpret their bodily states, seek care, and fashion themselves according to prevailing moral notions" (Nguyen and Peschard 2003:459). The effect of this systematic constrained agency is a type of violence that ultimately kills people through neglect (Galtung 1969; Farmer 1999, 2003; Foucault 2003).

Although negative representations and the practice of structural violence are persistent in the biopolitics of Hawaiian health, the exercise of power is not unidirectional. In examining the power relations exercised through the production of health, we can expect to find resistance (Foucault 1977 [1995]). Thus, Native Hawaiians' own views on how they came to be represented as unhealthy focus directly on the historical and social relations that have contributed to their contemporary disease burden (e.g., Blaisdell 1989, 1993). In fact, most accounts of the decline of Hawaiians' health begin with the arrival of Captain Cook in 1778. The diseases brought by Cook and his crew were the first of many to follow and by 1878 approximately 90 percent of the Hawaiian population had died (Stannard 1989). This startling depopulation is a potent reminder that the poor health of contemporary Hawaiians is not a new phenomenon, but is a consequence of their relationship with Europe and the United States.

The incorporation of the effects of medicalization, and the political economy through Native Hawaiians' understanding and experience of health reflects key issues in critical medical anthropology (Morsy 1996; Singer 2003). In the present research I found that narratives of "health" in contemporary Hawai'i are embedded in historical and social relations between Hawai'i and the West.[5] For many Native Hawaiians, health and what it means to achieve it become intertwined with ideas about who they are and their ability to maintain Hawaiian culture and their life. Among the participants of this work, definitions of health were embedded in ideas of what it means to be a Native Hawaiian and of their cultural and material dispossession. In remembering the lives, health, and subsequent dispossession of their ancestors, contemporary Hawaiians turn to alternative definitions of what it means to be a "healthy Hawaiian," raising questions about "health" as defined by biomedicine.

Accounting for the political economy of health illuminates what would otherwise be a naturalized conception of health that would be applied to overly decontextualized and medicalized individuals. In order to recontextualize Hawaiian health the following sections will tease out different structural factors that impact views and practices of health. These structural factors include loss of land and cultural independence and biomedicalization. Chapter 1 will address the historical structural factors related to political subordination and poverty that have constrained indigenous agency. Then, by focusing on the revitalization of identity this work integrates the local meanings with the historical and contemporary processes that facilitate opportunities for healthy living for some and constrain options for others. The examination of health and identity leads us to the embodied experience of Native Hawaiians themselves as actors remembering knowledge that was silenced, creating and engaging in potential moments of resistance, and taking "pragmatic action" (Lock 1993).

Biomedicalization—Defining Health

Framing the concept of health and a healthy body as fluid as well as culturally and historically contingent reveals the extent to which we have focused on a functional definition of health (Baer, Singer, and Susser 2003) and allowed the decontextualized meaning of health to remain unquestioned. Often the de facto definition of health is the absence of disease and the restoration of the body to a "normal" state of functioning. Health is defined in the negative sense; we do not think about the meaning of good health except when we do not have it (Canguilhem 1966 [1991]; Osborne 1997).

The process of retuning the body to "normality" has also been viewed as a site for the exercise of power by those who promote and those who use technologies of health (such as discourses of sanitation and hygiene, medicinals, and health clubs) (e.g., Foucault 1973, 1977 [1995]; Crandon-Malamud 1991; Crawford 1994; Brodwin 1996; Lupton 1997; Briggs and Mantini-Briggs 2003; Anderson 2006). Still, in order to observe the use of health technologies, the concept of health must be meaningful. Typically, in the practice and use of biomedicine, health is meaningful because it is taken as a fact based in biology (Foucault 1988; Osborne 1997). Consequently, as discussed in the previous section, we are left with an absurd tautology. If health is a biological given, then those who do not *have* health or populations who carry a greater burden of disease are said to be biologically different in either their genetic or civilizing abilities. These individuals and groups are thought to be *at risk* for an assortment of ailments that must be managed through governmental policies and technologies (Foucault 1977 [1995]; Lupton 1999; Nguyen and Peschard 2003, Castro and Singer 2004). In other words, the use of diagnostic tools in the exercise of knowledge/power or the choice of one medicinal over another as a statement of affiliation can be framed as either good or bad because health is taken to be a measurable biological fact (Foucault 1988). If we can only know health by its absence, then what is being measured when we say one is healthy?

Crawford (1984, 1994) is among the few scholars to closely examine the relationship between meanings of health and cultural identity. Drawing on Foucault, Crawford offers a history of the particular links between meanings of health and identity that are rooted in Enlightenment thought by noting:

> When the body became an abstracted entity, identical to all other bodies, detached from living situations, health became a concept for describing its normal state. The description became the goal: the restoration or maintaining of normal functioning. Thus, in unlocking the secrets of the body, medical science claimed to have discovered the laws of health. These laws were to be subjected to manipulation on behalf of the humanistic goals of the Enlightenment—the extension of life and the elimination of suffering. (1994:1350)

This line of thinking has two implications: firstly, in the effort to achieve the goal of good health, which is defined as the restoration and maintenance of the "normal" body, people become subject to new disciplinary techniques that will ensure normality—the "laws of health" (e.g., Canguilhem 1966; Foucault

1973, 1977 [1995]). The focus on lifestyle behaviors in public health (e.g., food pyramids, accounting for hours of exercise per week) is one example of this effort. Secondly, as the body is lifted out of context, "detached from its living situations," what is healthy for one is seen as healthy for all (an equality imbued by nature). As a result, the effects of social context on definitions of health become obscured and biomedical concepts and measures take precedence. Given the legitimacy and social standing of biomedicine in the United States and the symbolic force of concepts such as independence, productivity, and self-control, it is no surprise that most middle-class Americans define health reductively as "the body without disease." These concepts are tied to the notion that anyone can achieve health through self-discipline—a nutritious diet, exercise, and preventive medical care—regardless of the political and economic factors that frame their very existence (McMullin 2005; Singer and Baer 2007). This observation is significant because it not only reveals the practices used to legitimize scientific understandings and their link to knowledge/power, but also the internalization of knowledge into symbols of what it means to organize and participate in U.S. society as an independent and productive member.

Crawford also argues that situating health in these terms provides a marker for those who are "unhealthy" or diseased. His examination of meanings of health and their link to representation and identity provide another avenue through which we can understand how the taken-for-granted meaning of health is used to reinforce social processes and inequalities. Using health to represent the achieved goals of American society has "become a primary means of signification by which borders are maintained, threats, specified, and internal weaknesses shored up (Crawford 1994:1348)." Thus, the model of health becomes a signifier for successful membership in U.S. society. In contrast, the diseased body can be seen as a manifestation of the failure to practice those values associated with health, such as self-control, independence, and productivity; the "unhealthy" other is stigmatized and feared. Examining how concepts of health serve to maintain "normality" both at the level of the individual body and in society leads Crawford (1994) and others (Das 1990; Adelson 2000; McMullin 2005) to ask if such a notion of "health" is truly healthy. As Das noted: "We have to see how we may define health so that instead of becoming a measure of the normal and the pathological, a means by which power may be exercised upon the one who declares that he is in pain, it becomes a means for the practices of freedom" (1990:43). My argument (McMullin 2005), which is elaborated in Chapter 5, demonstrates that Native Hawaiian definitions of health do provide an alternative meaning of health. More importantly, these definitions are deeply intertwined with Hawaiian sovereignty and put into the service of promoting that sovereignty. As such, they reject representations of health as solely the result of biology, productivity, and individualism (Chapter 6). I do not, however, want to read Hawaiian knowledge as solely an act of Foucauldian resistance to the hegemonies of biomedicine. Rather, it is more useful to remember that health has potential for pragmatic action and resistance because, in its counter-hegemonic framing, it questions who has the power to determine what constitutes health. Moreover, this summary of capitalist meanings of health provides a framework from which to better understand the struggles and subjectivities of off-islanders who imbue mālama 'āina with a different potential.

Cultural Identity

Cultural identity has been a topic of great interest to scholars working on the Pacific. This is due, in part, to the ongoing decolonization of the Pacific and the relatively recent sovereignty regained by many island nations. The political autonomy regained by many of the islands raises questions about how Islanders revitalize and re-present their ideological and material culture. Renewed interest in reviving the knowledge and practices of our Pacific ancestors who struggled to survive under Western hegemony both empowers contemporary islanders as well as poses new challenges for the meaning of health within concepts of culture, place, and identity.

Previous debates about identity, its relationship to politics, nationalism, and culture have typically used ethnicity as an explanatory concept. An ethnic identity is seen as highly politicized and necessary in a time of struggles for power and resources. When drawing on an ethnic identity, a group emphasizes exclusion of others in the hope of creating greater unification within the group (Barth 1969; Comaroff 1987; Gilroy 1990; Linnekin and Poyer 1990). Ethnicity has been a continual source for the creation of boundaries and their maintenance through cultural differentiation (Barth 1969). Although the creation and maintenance of boundaries describes part of the processes associated with identity, it leaves little room to engage the fluidity of identity.

An ongoing debate in defining ethnic, cultural, and national identities has revolved around avoiding the creation of static categories and disputes of authenticity[6] (Brown 2004). Part of the struggle is to simultaneously recognize indigenous meanings and the shifting nature of identities (Morton Lee 2003). As islanders are increasing efforts to maintain or revive the ways of their ancestors, they are also contesting the culture of their colonizers, and the hegemonic identities that are a consequence of colonization (Friedman 1994). Subsequently, belonging to a group that emphasizes both the inequalities produced through colonization, economic transformations, and contemporary alternatives based on the remembrance of their ancestors reinforces the importance of defining identity as a fluid or unfolding process. Thus, when Linnekin and Poyer state that studies of cultural identities are "concerned with the cultural dimensions of identity; that is with symbols, meanings and indigenous categories" (1990:4) or Hall states that cultural identities are "those aspects of our identities which arise from our 'belonging' to distinctive ethnic, racial, linguistic, religious, and above all national cultures" (Hall 1996:596) they are mediating key aspects of identity making and embodiment in political contexts.

A final point where anthropologists have contested static definitions of identity is in its association with race. Howard (1990) and more recently Kauanui (2008) note clear differences between Western colonial and Pacific Island concepts of identity. Whereas colonial concepts of identity focus on the primacy of race and genetics, Pacific concepts of identity often emphasize the maintenance of relations with community and land that are ultimately infused with genealogical connections. Therefore, one's identity is represented by social networks and the consumption of food that is obtained from the land of one's ancestors. Failure to maintain connections with family, friends, and land results in a transformation of social relationships that negates a claim to a particular island identity and the links associated with one's current networks and location. For example, Poyer's 1993 study of a small Micronesian atoll (Ngatik, also known as Sapwuahfik) examines the historical contingency of a Sapwuahfik identity through the emphasis on relations and behavior and the de-emphasis of genetic ties to that identity. The near-complete genocide of the Sapwuahfik population by the crew of a merchant ship searching for tortoise shell in the 1800s instigated a rethinking of their island identity. Despite the fact that crew members of the merchant ship (Pohnpeians, Marshallese, other Pacific Islanders, and Americans) all contributed to the repopulation of Sapwuahfik, the renewed identity was not based on exclusion of migrant groups, but rather on inclusion based on shared performances of everyday life, such as consumption of food, mannerisms, genealogical ties, and remaining socially connected to relatives on-island. Furthermore, the massacre became a significant shared historical event that contributes to the meaning of contemporary Sapwuahfik identity. In this case the revitalization of a cultural identity entails an emphasis on practices, not on specific blood ties to the indigenous people of the island.

In terms of issues of identity in Hawai'i, the depopulation of Natives from the islands and the influx of migrant workers brought by colonists have some similarities with Sapwuahfik. Behavior, maintaining relationships with family and friends, and genealogical ties to the islands are important factors as they are for most Pacific Islanders.[7] Yet, the role of the U.S. government in defining what is meant by genealogical ties and the political implications of that definition have structured much of the historical dispossession of Hawaiians from the 'āina (the land and genealogical ancestor). Most institutions, from sovereignty groups to the U.S. government, accept the statement that anyone who has ties to pre-contact (before the arrival of Captain Cook in 1778) Hawaiians is considered a Native Hawaiian. The U.S. government, however, has continually shifted the legal definition of this identity based on genetic inheritance, from tracing the lineage through the maternal to the paternal ancestors and shifting the "blood quantum" necessary to be considered a Native (Linnekin 1983; Kauanui 2008). The significance of the blood quantum relationship to pre-contact Hawaiians is linked to the U.S. requirements that allow Native Hawaiians to have access to land and other social and economic resources on the islands. For example, Native Hawaiians must prove they have at least 50 percent Hawaiian blood quantum to apply to the waiting list for Hawaiian Homes Land. In contrast to the criteria enforced by the U.S. government, some Native Hawaiian groups say that people who can trace *any* percentage of their ancestry to pre-contact Hawaiians should be included on this list. Identifying oneself as Native Hawaiian then, is not simply about affiliation with a body of knowledge and a set of practices, it is a political statement about who can and cannot have access to resources. Native Hawaiian or Kanaka Maoli[8] identity is historically, politically, and behaviorally contingent and fluid. As Kauanui (2008) argues, the imposition of these federal laws has adversely affected both the historical conceptions of kinship and identity as well as Kanaka Maoli efforts to regain sovereignty over the islands.

The contingency of identity also raises questions about how Hawaiians living off-island represent themselves. Participation in Hawaiian activities such as hula, language, and festivals is one of the more prominent ways to embody the ancestors' knowledge and create a sense of community. Like on-islanders, the ability to claim an ancestral heritage is also increasingly important to identifying oneself as a Native Hawaiian (Kauanui 2000; Halualani 2002), particularly in light of off-island civic clubs' active inclusion of non-Hawaiians or "Hawaiians at Heart." Kauanui (2007) has argued that the overemphasis on off-islander practices such as hula and lu'au (practices that are inextricably intertwined with tourism and are attractive to many non-Hawaiians) promotes the erasure of Hawaiians' long history of migration, and political and economic participation on the west coast of the continent. Kauanui notes that the combination of non-Hawaiians engaging in "Hawaiian" practices and the forgetting of their migration history (from the 1800s and probably earlier), leads to characterizations of off-islanders who do not practice hula or speak Hawaiian as not "real" Hawaiians (Kauanui 2007:154). While off-islander identity is not as politically linked to issues of access to land like their counterparts back home, their "Hawaiian-ness" is still subject to the desires and definitions of others. Understanding the ways that off-islanders experience "Hawaiianness" in relation to practices, genealogical ties, and land provides insight into the fluidity of identity and health.

The fluidity of identity is reflected in Hall's argument that cultural identity is always in a state of "becoming" (Hall 1994). For instance, he argues that:

Perhaps instead of thinking of identity as an already accomplished fact, which the new cultural practices then represent, we should think, instead, of identity as a "production", which is never complete, always in process, and always constituted within, not outside, representation (1994:392).

The representations that are used to claim a particular cultural identity whether from popular culture or from representations of health are not static, "we all write and speak from a particular place and time, from a history and a culture which is specific. What we say is always 'in context', *positioned* (Hall 1994:392, emphasis in original)." Cultural identity as it is revitalized by contemporary Native Hawaiians reveals a position in relation to ancestors, missionaries, colonizers, current struggles with hegemony, and future goals. In turn, Native Hawaiians living off-island have had a somewhat different experience with the revitalization efforts than those who have stayed "at home." In both cases, however, thinking of cultural identity as being constituted from within the experiences of the speaker allows us to examine how identity is in a state of "becoming," rather than something fixed and immutable. Thus, an examination of representations and individual experiences of cultural identity as they are expressed in concepts of health pushes us to interrogate the fluidity of the healthy body and the processes by which inequality and poor health are produced or maintained.

Loss of Land and Cultural Independence: History, Sovereignty, and Identity

My research was conducted during a time of concerted efforts towards charting positive directions for Native Hawaiians through the decolonization of Hawaiian land and through the revitalization of material and non-material culture. Over the last few decades increasingly cohesive groups of Native Hawaiians have made concerted efforts to "decolonize the minds" of their people, to bring back the knowledge, and lifestyles of their ancestors (Kanahele 1986; Trask 1993). Many Native Hawaiians, both at the grassroots and institutional level, decided that it was time to stop the decline of Hawaiian culture and pride. It was time to regroup, look to the kūpuna (the elders) as a source of knowledge for the restoration of Hawaiian culture. This renaissance has not been confined to material and non-material culture. It is also a part of a political movement aimed at improving the economic situation of Native Hawaiians and their access to land. In other words, the movement's ultimate goal is cultural and economic independence for Native Hawaiians. These efforts include increasing numbers of hula hālau (hula schools), the flourishing of Punana Leo (Hawaiian language immersion schools), voyages of the vessel Hokuleʻa,[9] use of traditional healing methods, and restoration of kalo gardens and fish ponds.

While efforts to restore practices such as hula, language, and voyaging have flourished, regaining control of land continues to be problematic. Similar to their history of health, Hawaiians have been engaged in constant struggles over land and sovereignty (e.g., Silva 2004). As will be discussed in more detail in Chapter 1, a significant event leading to the disenfranchisement of Native Hawaiians from their land is the 1848 Māhele (division). The Māhele transformed the traditional communal land tenure system to private ownership.[10] Thus, many Hawaiians lost control of and access to the land on which their families had lived and worked for generations. Kameʻeleihiwa (1992) argues that the culmination of these transformations of land "ownership" was the illegal overthrow of the Hawaiian monarchy. In January of 1893, Queen Liliʻuokalani's monarchy was deposed, and the queen was placed under house arrest by a group of American businessmen and planters, supported by the U.S. military.[11] Although President Cleveland (1893, House Ex. Doc 47) refused to lay claim to the Hawaiian Islands, his successor, President McKinley, held a pro-annexation position, and in 1898 the Hawaiian Islands were made a U.S. territory and ultimately became the fiftieth state in 1959.

One hundred years after the illegal overthrow, the U.S. Congress apologized on behalf of the United States for its actions against the kingdom of Hawaiʻi (1993 P.L. 103–150). Most revealing, perhaps, is the disclaimer contained within the apology: "Nothing in this Joint Resolution is intended to serve as a settlement of any claims against the United States." While the United States was willing to recognize the illegality of their actions, repatriation of Native Hawaiians to the land remains a goal yet to be achieved.

Contemporary struggles to restore Hawaiian land and political independence can be seen through the activities of the various sovereignty movements. The primary goal of sovereignty is the restoration of a Hawaiian land base and the right to self-governance. The movements vary in the type of relationship they envision having with the United States. They range from the establishment of a nation-within-a-nation, modeled after Native American Indians, to a free association, or a complete secession from the United States. These movements, however, are complicated by a lack of federal recognition as an indigenous people. As a consequence the welfare of the Native Hawaiian people has been placed in the State Office of Hawaiian Affairs (OHA), which administers programs designed to benefit Native Hawaiians. Kauanui (2002) has outlined many problems with federal recognition: that recognition would concede Native Hawaiian's citizenship within the United States, it would allow the United States to define who is and is not Hawaiian through blood quantum levels, and it would provide symbolic weight to the vote that made Hawai'i the fiftieth state. Due to the illegal overthrow of the Monarchy, it is also assumed that the vote to become the fiftieth state is also illegal and thus invalid. If Native Hawaiians acquire federal recognition, then that finding will be used as an indication that they also recognize the authority of the United States to make Hawai'i a state. Lack of federal recognition, however, has also led to the recent court decision where (in Rice v. Cayetano (98–818) 146 F.3d 1075 reversed), the United States Supreme Court (February 23, 2000) found that denying Rice, a resident of Hawai'i, the right to vote in the OHA elections violated the Fifteenth Amendment. The court found that it was racially discriminatory to prohibit non-Hawaiians to vote in the statewide elections for OHA trustees, whose role it is to oversee the welfare of Native Hawaiians. The contested nature of Hawaiian citizenship, and its political and economic link to land and cultural knowledge, can be reflected in the larger social discourse on Native Hawaiian health.

Nationalism

The current renaissance and nationalist movements in Hawai'i provide a mechanism through which a Native Hawaiian past and potential future are envisioned. Theories of nationalism, like theories of ethnicity, address issues dealing with the homogenization of beliefs and the exclusion of other beliefs and people. As Handler (1988) argues, a primary goal of nationalist movements is to "homogenize the diversity of everyday life." Homogenization often takes place through the establishment of tradition, continuity with the past through which a community can "imagine" its similarities (Anderson 1991 [1983]).

According to Anderson (1991 [1983]), individuals in a community imagine that they have shared experiences and similar goals and desires, which creates a shared bond of nationalism. A return to tradition and history plays a large role in reconstructing a past, a shared history, and a means by which to imagine a community and interpret the present. The legacy of colonialism and its ramifications bind many current nationalist movements (Linnekin and Poyer 1990; Friedman 1994; Hereniko 1994). Nationalist movements emphasize creating a group of people who share not only artifacts, rituals, and symbols, but also a particular view of life that is represented through the experiences of their ancestors.

One aspect of nation building concerns culture and the use of tradition. Anderson (1991 [1983]) argues that one of the key consequences of printed material on national consciousness was that it "gave a new fixity to language, which in the long run helped to build that image of antiquity so central to the subjective idea of the nation." The image of antiquity is important because it provides a means to establish continuity with the past (Hobsbawm and Ranger 1983). The Hawaiian renaissance and sovereignty movement began as grassroots efforts (see Trask 1983, 1993, 1994). The members of these movements strive to have Hawaiian language immersion schools and create greater access to Hawaiian knowledge, that is, books, dances, chants, land. Renaissance and sovereignty movements have organized these efforts, and have incorporated traditional knowledge from these grassroots organizations, lay people, and other Pacific scholars into their writings, which can then be used to reconstitute a foundation of Native Hawaiian knowledge. The emphasis is on creating a group of people who have and share not only a history, but also a particular cultural view of life that embodies the norms and values of their ancestors. Thus, the use of tradition is intermixed with issues of cultural identity and nationalism. As Friedman (1994) has noted, it is the dehegemonization of Western ideals that has created the context in which these movements are able to rise, return to their traditions, and imagine themselves as one.

The idea of an imagined community, a community in which each member does not necessarily know every other member, but nevertheless has a sense of sharing in the struggle for the same objectives, beliefs, and way of life allows us to view culture and the movement of people in new ways, reflecting the fluidity of identity. Since some scholars have argued that cultural meaning systems reside in the minds and actions of people, that is, not in the land from which the people came, new debates over the place of culture, and transnational culture flows have emerged. These debates highlight complicated processes that produce both an essentialized view of identity as "the blood" as well as the conflation inequality and culture that is manifested in poor health.

Transnational Inscriptions of Place and Body

An important theoretical aspect in the reconstruction of a Native Hawaiian cultural identity and ideology is the emphasis on their roots emerging from a specific geographic location and the need to repopulate the islands with more Native Hawaiians. We do not typically think of Native Hawaiians as a diasporic community nor view those who live off island as "transnationals." Yet, the Hawaiian archipelago represents a spatial location that marks the boundaries of the Hawaiian nation. The Hawaiian nation is conceptualized both as a politically bounded location and as the people who, according to the goals of the Hawaiian renaissance and sovereignty, should be occupying that space. The Hawaiian Islands are a geographical location that represents historical, social, and moral ideals that provide significant motivational force for the improvement of the physical and spiritual well-being of Hawaiian land and bodies. These details position off-islanders as people who have migrated across national borders and who are subject to processes that affect diasporic peoples. As Spickard (2002) notes, a transnational/diasporic understanding of Pacific Islander migration best describes the experience of migration as these populations generally do not assimilate into the dominant population, nor do they subscribe to a Pacific pan-ethnic identity.

A key interest of transnational researchers is how migrants maintain political and cultural identity in their new home in relation to their homeland. Migrants must often negotiate the hegemonic discourses, such as biomedicine, coming from both nations (Basch et al. 1994). As Gupta (1992) has argued, the process of negotiating national hegemonies involves a "reinscription of space." As migrants live in a locale they create new connections and practices that in some ways mirror those in their nation of origin. It is transmigrants' ability to live, to reinscribe their local environment, yet remain rooted in their homeland that has been of interest to many researchers. Although transmigrants do not physically occupy their home nation, they often remain socially, culturally, and economically tied to it (Rouse 1991; Gupta 1992; Basch et al. 1994; Kearney 1995). Migrants' continuing relationship with their home nation results in a deterritorialization of the nation. As Gupta and Ferguson (1992) have noted, it is the deterritorialization of space that has forced us to deal with ideas of cultural difference, while complicating the notion of localized culture. For example, anthropologists examining cultural processes must not be constrained by the geographical location of the Hawaiian archipelago, and yet because of the historical and current cultural and political importance of the land we must take into account the shift in associated meanings. Deterritorialization, increased globalization, and an imagined community facilitate cultural flows, making Native Hawaiian meaning systems possible anywhere. And if Native Hawaiian culture is possible anywhere, what symbols give rise to emerging imagined communities?

Following the work of Stuart Hall, Gupta and Ferguson (1992) have argued that identity must be viewed as a "meeting point"—a point of suture—that constitutes and re-forms the subject so as to enable that subject to act. The emphasis on the relational aspects in this conceptualization of identity is appropriate for Native Hawaiians in California as they live in a context that emphasizes control and independence through fit bodies de-linked from place and history as a sign of health. Yet, off-islanders beautifully express their relationship with Hawaiian ancestors and their peers by attending festivals, practicing hula, and learning Hawaiian, among other things. This temporary "suturing" of identity through Hawaiian bodies that remember ancestors and capitalist bodies that are able to produce highlights the historical and political forces that impact transnational culture flows. Both capitalist and Hawaiian bodies have the potential to be healthy; however, they have very different political implications. Because the political importance of access to the land and of remembering ancestors through the land is not as viable in the cultural flows of transnational knowledge, the suturing occurs when healthy Hawaiian bodies are constructed through self-discipline and biomedicine. The resultant body that is disciplined through these technologies becomes a way to practice cultural identity; this "suturing" has a remainder—the genealogy of and struggle over the 'āina—for which there is no accounting. A healthy Hawaiian body that is linked to political struggle refracts the social fault lines where poor health and immiseration are fostered. If there is no accounting for the remainder we are left with the capitalist body, one that is ready to produce services, materials for consumption, and identities. The healthy capitalist body is ultimately attributable to the hegemony of biomedicine when transnational cultural flows do not incorporate histories of healthy and unhealthy Hawaiians. Without the inclusion of the historical and political context there is no robust alternative discourse to contest the pervasiveness of individual control and responsibility for health. Focusing on how healthy bodies are points of suture for identity issues unveils the way in which social struggles can slide into discourses of individual achievement—the opposite poles in debates over cultural meanings and political economies of health.

Imagining a community in which ties are maintained yet cultural differences are expressed impacts the decisions that transmigrants make about their identity and the spaces they occupy.[12] Basch et al. (1994) argued that transmigrants do not see themselves as a part of two nations, but rather form an identity that reflects the connections between the various nations that they have created for themselves. As such, understandings of land, food, health, and body take on shared and contradictory meanings that refract the historical, political, and structural processes that transnational Hawaiian communities face as they reinscribe place and find ways to embody their ancestors through a Native Hawaiian identity. These reconfigured meanings, however, can potentially diminish discourses of inequities produced by the political economy and experienced by on-islanders. Focusing on health as solely an issue of biology or identity individualizes and depoliticizes practices that remember ancestors, and it obscures the socio-political remembering of ancestors that insists on the association between land, health, and sovereignty.

Outline of Chapters

Responses to what it means to be a healthy Hawaiian throw into relief the fluidity, contestation, and suturing of existing ideals of health. More importantly the representations of health in Hawai'i reveal historical and contemporary political struggles that maintain and revitalize a Native Hawaiian cultural identity. This knowledge of health provides a framework for a counter-hegemonic discourse that reconfigures Enlightenment and biomedical discourses and practices. The following chapters examine the links between views of Native Hawaiian health that call attention to social and economic inequalities as they are intertwined with the land and the facets of variation for Native Hawaiians living on- or off-island (Hawai'i and California).

Chapter 1 presents a brief history of health in Hawai'i. Captain Cook and the foreigners who followed are viewed as the carriers of disease and as people filled with colonial desires. The staggering depopulation is framed not only as the effects of contact on a population who had little exposure to these infectious diseases, but also as a potential example of a syndemic (Singer and Clair 2003). Although these interactions were among the first threats to the health of Hawaiians by foreigners, they were not the last. Drawing from the research of historians, I outline the struggles of Native Hawaiians' incorporation of and resistance to the imposition of institutional structures associated with the practice of biomedicine and the maintenance of Hawaiian medical practices. These historical events frame attitudes towards Native Hawaiian health and medicinal practices as they become a point of contention not only in the struggle for land and cultural hegemony in the Islands but for the physical survival of the Hawaiian people. Finally, I discuss recent efforts to promote Hawaiian health such as the Wai'anae diet. Some of the contemporary efforts to restore health remind Hawaiians of the lifestyles of their ancestors, while simultaneously highlighting the political context that gave rise to their current health status. As such, these historical events provide a framework for a cultural memory that contextualizes current health inequalities and anchors the counter-hegemonic discourse in politics and identity.

Chapter 2 examines the complexities of conducting research in Hawai'i and with Native Hawaiians. The first part of this chapter discusses the cultural construction of Hawai'i as a research location and Native Hawaiians as a group that "have culture." Characterizations of the Hawaiian Islands as primarily a tourist destination and as the home of a population whose culture has been decimated by disease and capitalism are reverse sides of the same representation. One representation is intertwined with ideas of culture as static and the other is an erasure of historical inequalities. Both representations are achieved and maintained through romantic visions of Hawai'i as paradise. The second part of this chapter presents my methods and the field sites where I conducted this study. I explore the importance of the management of my identity both by those I lived and spoke with, and by myself. The events described in this chapter reveal the complicated relationship between my own identity and how I was perceived by others, which in the end, helped me gain partial understanding of key practices and understandings of health, identity, and inequality.

Chapter 3 is an examination of health care practices in Hawai'i and California. The documented poor health of the Hawaiian population resulted in a plethora of studies that attempted to answer questions of "non-compliance" among Hawaiians, which was typically characterized as a "failure" to seek biomedical care. Using data from my fieldwork in Hawai'i, I document economic and personal reasons Native Hawaiians give for not seeking care from biomedical practitioners. Understanding the reasons given for resisting care from biomedical practitioners highlights the complexities of overall health-seeking behaviors. These complexities entail searches for doctors who practice both biomedicine as well as Hawaiian medicine, mixing technological advances such as x-rays with care from traditional Hawaiian practitioners. Moreover, the complicating factors associated with seeking biomedical care, such as insurance forms, documentation of procedures, and generalized frustration with being the subject of medical questioning and research, suggest biopolitical attempts at normalization and integration into the capitalist system. The intersection of structural factors such as economics and access to new technologies, and individual issues such as learning from and being cared for by someone who is Native Hawaiian or at least who understands Hawaiian ways creates a contrast between decontextualized "Western" ways of practicing medicine and the contextualized "purity" of Hawaiian ways. This contrast also provides another level from which to understand health inequalities in terms of social spaces and the debate over medical knowledge. In contrast, health practices in California, while thought to be better, are constrained by the availability of practitioners of Hawaiian medicine. As a result, Californian Hawaiians' health care choices emphasize economic factors as primary barriers to care. This chapter argues that health-seeking can be a negotiation between physical, economic, and cultural needs rather than a representation of personal "failure" to seek "appropriate" care by Native Hawaiians. The debates and struggles to obtain medical care parallel the historical struggles to maintain the legitimacy of Hawaiian medical practices. As such, these structural processes refract social facets that influence the fluidity of identity and the meaning given to inequality between on- and off-islanders.

Chapter 4 is a comparative examination of competing definitions of health and their salience for the cultural memory of Native Hawaiians. In this chapter I examine variations in how health is used as a symbol to define what it means to be a Native Hawaiian and, more importantly, a healthy Native Hawaiian. Health is used both as an inclusionary and exclusionary category. As an exclusionary category, "haole" behaviors (past and present) provide an image against which Native Hawaiians define themselves and, as in the health-seeking chapter, explain inequality. The experiences of Hawaiians in California result in a cultural memory that can be traced to the health of Hawaiians when they left the islands, rather than to pre-contact ancestors. The emphasis on biomedicine and preventive lifestyle behaviors as defined by public health and popular media provide the context for understanding health off-island. In contrast, a "traditional" Hawaiian lifestyle is used to define what and how Hawaiians were and can be in the future. In examining the general meaning of health we see how Native Hawaiian cultural identities and alternative discourses can be positioned in contrast to colonizers, biomedicine, as well as in contrast to their counterparts on- or off-island.

Chapter 5 furthers our understanding of health by examining specific elements that are stated as necessary to being a healthy Hawaiian. The elements used are contextual categories that allow us to elaborate on the significance of health in the production of a counter-hegemonic discourse and the formation of cultural identity. The understanding of health developed here is layered by questioning the portability of meanings attributed to symbols of health among transnational communities. There are three intersecting themes that are used to create an image of Hawaiian health. The first theme, access to land, intimately links issues of food and social relationships. The land where Hawaiian ancestors lived is imbued with mana, a life force that restores physical and spiritual balance. Moreover, kalo is a cornerstone of the Hawaiian diet. Thus, Hawaiian land links relationships to the ancestors, contemporary Hawaiians, and health through food that comes from the land. The shift in land ownership and access to land for both subsistence and communal purposes creates the highly contentious and political struggles over both Hawaiian sovereignty and health. The second theme is that of food. The introduction of Western foods resulted in Hawaiians eating foods that caused disease. Hawaiian foods, in contrast are healthier and natural. These themes reflect the importance of history and land in the revitalization of Hawaiian health knowledge, which culminate in the third theme, the image of the "Healthy Ancestor." The Healthy Ancestor serves as a potent metaphor both as a guide for achieving a healthy state and as an image of Hawaiian cultural identity. This ancestor is the embodiment of Native Hawaiians' struggle. While the Healthy Ancestor was a prominent link between food and land, for Hawaiians in California being a healthy Hawaiian was achieved through the link of food and body, which allowed you to live as a Hawaiian and to practice the symbols of Hawaiian identity such as hula, language, music, and festivals. Technology has enhanced the ability of transnational communities to maintain links and weave the symbols of their homeland with their experiences in their new place of residence. Yet, some symbols and cultural models, such as health, may not take on the same meaning or motivational force as they do in the islands. This analysis reveals the importance of context in the struggle over the meaning of models of health and shows that some cultural symbols are not as portable (land) as other cultural symbols (hula) and yet both give rise to a particular kind of remembering of ancestors and achieving health.

In Chapter 6 I examine the impact that transformations in access to Hawaiian land and food have had on redefining the body. While the Healthy Ancestor provides an embodied image of a healthy Hawaiian, the fit, lean body has long been viewed as the product of intense control underpinned by capitalist ideology. The categorization of obesity as a disease furthers this argument by situating the large body as pathological, as a symbol of an inability to control desires, and as the failure of a productive body. These images of the body also represent the implicit link between body size and meanings of physical health. This hegemonic understanding of body and health obscures alternative meanings of both large bodies and fit, lean bodies. In the Pacific Islands large bodies are often viewed as a sign of social health, that others care for you. More recently, the fit, lean body also has an alternative meaning that is politicized within the framework of social and physical health; a fit lean body that is linked to the well-being of ancestors, and is prevented first by colonialism, and then capitalism and globalization. I trace the shifts in the meaning of the body as it is linked to categories of health and pathology, lean and obese. I argue that in those moments when the fit, lean Native Hawaiian body is used to contest hegemonic ideology, the political struggles of Native Hawaiians are brought to the fore and inequalities are highlighted. It is at this moment, however, that the Native Hawaiian healthy body is also made vulnerable to biopolitics and hegemonic reinterpretations that seek to show a controlled, productive, and disciplined body.

The final chapter examines the centrality of health in the revitalization of cultural identity and as a counter-hegemonic movement. Because health is part of daily life, the models used to represent health, or the lack thereof, give insight into the ongoing political struggles. I argue that a critical medical anthropology approach that focuses attention on the meaning of health as a reflection of issues of cultural identity allows us to see how power relationships that create individual knowledge and deny social knowledge of health are obscured. Transnationalism and globalization complicate efforts to transform health practices through the insistence on a mobile, generic body that can be traced back to Enlightenment views of health. Thus, the alternative/counter-hegemonic health discourse that Native Hawaiians push for must constantly attend to the slippage between health and its representations as natural. A focus on the political economy and its inequities must be maintained. In the struggles to regain Hawaiian sovereignty, health is the embodiment of the inequalities experienced by Native Hawaiians. As such, highlighting alternative definitions of health that affirm Native Hawaiian identity and practices, provides a positive direction for Hawaiians and points to the fact that poor health is not natural, but rather the product of unequal social forces.

Endnotes

1. Rates for circulatory disease 415 per 100,000, cancer 231 per 100,000 (Johnson, Oyama, and Marchand 1998).
2. Age-adjusted morbidity rates for Native Hawaiians, three-year average, 1989–1991. Rates per 100,000. Hypertension 97.7, asthma 74.4, diabetes 39.5. (Health Surveillance Program, Office of Health Status Monitoring, Hawaii State Department of Health. Johnson, Oyama, and Marchand 1998:303).
3. See Howard (1974) for a more thorough account of how his research group was chosen to conduct work with Hawaiians and an overview of the many studies produced through his research agenda. After the Lili'uokalani Trust (1962) conducted a survey documenting many concerns for the Hawaiian community, Howard was approached by the Lili'uokalani research committee and the Bishop Museum to conduct research with the Hawaiian community in order to better understand the cultural processes that give rise to their being "overrepresented in virtually all categories of 'social problems'"(ix). Howard and his research group conducted ethnographic examinations of the daily lives of Hawaiians, including family life, alcohol consumption, education, and health. Gallimore (1974), also part of the research group, conducted the psychological components of the study, particularly as they applied to youth and education.
4. The work of other scholars of colonialism in Africa and Latin American also reports similar techniques of control and processes of civilization (cf. Comaroff 1985; Briggs and Mantini-Briggs 2003).
5. Though Hawai'i is west of the continental United States, I am using the term to signify ideologies associated with Euro-American expansion across the Pacific. See Trouillot 2003 for a more critical discussion on the use of the "West."
6. Studies of ethnic identity, additionally, suffer from a tendency to question the authenticity of identity (Linnekin and Poyer 1990; Friedman 1994; Briggs 1996). The symbols that are used to create the bond among people in a particular ethnic group are continually called into question. This issue stems from the literature on the invention of tradition (e.g., Hobsbawm and Ranger 1983). For example, Linnekin (1983), in her work on the concept of mālama 'āina (caring for the land), asserts that this symbol was created in order to bring an image of unity among Hawaiians, which would then assist them in their current political and economic struggles. Many Hawaiians took offense over the assertion that this was a recent invention (e.g., Trask 1993; Kame'eleihiwa 1992). Keesing (1989) also argued that many symbols used by Native activists were merely used for political advantage and were not part of the lived experiences of Islanders. Keesing engaged in a contentious debate with Trask (1991) over the authority that anthropologists use to negate the "existence" of specific symbols in island history. For Trask (1991), determining the "authenticity" of symbols speaks to the issue of anthropologists having more power to define Hawaiian identity than Hawaiians themselves. In reasserting their power to speak for themselves, Hawaiian scholars have shown through their own research

the historical importance of mālama 'āina and other significant cultural concepts and their ties to pre-contact Hawaiians.

7. Behavior also plays a significant role in defining "Hawaiianness." For example, one may hear a Native Hawaiian referred to as a *haole* for exhibiting behavior attributed to white people (typically being stingy, arrogant or too inquisitive), or you may hear non-Natives or locals (people who have lived in Hawai'i for significant amounts of time) referred to as "Hawaiians at heart" because of their typically "Hawaiian" behavior. In other words, a Native Hawaiian may be excluded from the group, or a non-Native may be included in the group because of their behavior; the non-Native however, would not be considered a "Native Hawaiian," but rather a "Hawaiian at heart." In addition many Native Hawaiians take great offense if someone who merely resides in Hawai'i, and does not have any Hawaiian ancestry, refers to himself as a Hawaiian.

8. Kanaka Maoli means real or true person. Kanaka means person, maoli true or real. Kanaka Maoli is gaining in use among Hawaiian scholars as it is the older term for Native Hawaiians who share linguistic relationships with other Oceanic peoples (Silva 2004).

9. See Chapter 1 for more detail on the Hawaiian language immersion programs and the Hokule'a.

10. Kame'eleihiwa (1992) argues that the Ali'i, when they agreed to the Māhele, believed that they were sharing the land or 'Āina with the people and not creating private ownership. This is based on two issues, one being the word *māhele* also means *to share*. The second issue is that the 'Āina could only be owned by the Gods, the Akua, and the 'Āina was in essence an Akua. Therefore no one could own an Akua and thus no one could own the land.

11. The following historical information is summarized from Trask 1993, and Kuykendall 1966. The group of businessmen sought to further secure their sugar interests at a time when Queen Lili'uokalani was attempting to ratify a new constitution that would remove the increasing amount of influence Americans had in her government and over the Hawaiian people. These businessmen viewed Lili'uokalani's actions as a threat to their interests. At the urging of the American Minister to Hawai'i, John L. Stevens, whose interests were aligned with the businessmen, the U.S. military was persuaded to land troops in Honolulu. With the landing of the troops the American group quickly set up what they called the Provisional Government, which was then officially recognized by Minister Stevens. It was under this military pressure that Queen Lili'uokalani ceded her authority to the United States government, not the Provisional Government. It was the Queen's hope that the United States government would recognize the injustices that had occurred and return control of the islands to the Hawaiian kingdom.

The Cleveland administration refused to recognize the Provisional Government and further refused to annex the Hawaiian Islands. With the change in the administration in 1897, however, and President McKinley's pro-annexation position, neither the Queen nor the stolen lands (1,800,000 acres of crown lands) were ever restored. In 1898, the Hawaiian Islands were annexed, and ultimately made the 50th state in 1959. For further historical/political works see Trask 1993; Kame'eleihiwa 1992; Kent 1993; Dougherty 1992.

12. The imagination of a community or nation does not come about by simply believing that it exists. History, politics, and social institutions provide contexts and mechanisms for building a nation and imagining that community. The belief in a shared

history is an important legitimating and psychological factor in the establishment of a nation (Hobsbawm and Ranger 1983; Anderson 1991 [1983]; Holland 1992; Friedman 1994). A sense of shared history brings about notions of rights to inhabit specific territories, and an innate biological birth right to make decisions concerning a geographic area (Anderson 1983; Hobsbawm and Ranger 1983; Linnekin 1992; Balibar and Wallerstein 1991; Basch et al. 1994). In addition, social institutions such as schools and bureaucracies add to the building of nations. The ability of schools to enculturate children through a national language and history provides the building blocks of shared experiences and beliefs among people. Finally, bureaucracies ensure the implementation and reification of laws that represent the values and morals of the nation or community (Handler 1988; Gupta 1992; Basch et al. 1994).

1

HAWAIIAN HEALTH: A CASUALTY OF HISTORY

Ideas about health in the Hawaiian context are framed by historical events such as contact with Europeans and Americans, depopulation, colonization, and resistance.[1] The familiar concepts of a "healthy Hawaiian body" and its counterpart the "unhealthy Hawaiian body" in conversations about Native Hawaiians create potent symbols for the renaissance and sovereignty movements. It is not simply, however, that these images are symbols of current efforts at self-determination. Rather, the body and health are an integral part of how Native Hawaiians can conceptualize social relationships with each other and their land base. Anderson notes that, "nationalism has to be understood by aligning it, not with self-consciously held political ideologies, but with the large cultural systems that preceded it, out of which—as well as against which—it came into being (1991 [1983]:12)." Historical and contemporary understandings of health are indeed a part of the "large cultural systems" within which Hawaiian nationalism is understood. Talking about health in a national context serves a dual purpose: it allows us to conceptualize it as a state of being everyone experiences as an individual and, when defined by normalizing effects of scientific knowledge or by local genealogical knowledge, as a population. Consequently, it follows that health is not only a political ideology but also part of a larger cultural system that connects individual and group as well as past and present. Examining the political facets of health leads to a denaturalization of healthy and unhealthy bodies, revealing the tensions and embodiments of inequality and normalizing effects as experienced by Native Hawaiians.

While Friedman (1994) has noted that a key aspect of Hawaiian identity is defined in direct opposition to the ways of the Europeans and Americans. Hawaiians' return to their history, to understanding the knowledge and practices of their ancestors, brings into view the political economy of health that produced transformations in social structure, knowledge and the physical well-being of so many. As we explore how Native Hawaiians remember the health of their ancestors it can be argued that identity is not simply a rejection of aspects of modernity and American colonialism, but rather an opportunity to remember shared histories and put forth other Hawaiian subjectivities.

Many Native Hawaiians I spoke with and much of contemporary Hawaiian literature positions Hawaiians and constitutes their identity as a group through the shared understanding of indigenous history, which provides a counterpoint to dominant European and American ideologies. Anderson 1991 [1983] and others (Hobsbawm and Ranger 1983) have argued that the use of familiar aspects of a shared history is necessary in order to build a sense of commonality that recognizes the fluidity of identity and resists the fragmentation of identity in the face of a more dominant homogenizing history that suppresses Hawaiian knowledge. The hegemony of Western[2] history and ideologies is precisely what Native Hawaiians continue to struggle against. The ability to draw on their history to build national and cultural identity binds people together in the sense of sharing common experiences and also gives them an alternative history that can be used to fragment the dominant history of the West.

Contact with the Western world has clearly affected the health status of Hawaiians in dramatic ways. Explorers and later waves of immigrants brought diseases that contributed to the depopulation of Hawai'i. The introduction of Western medicine and efforts by missionaries to devalue Hawaiian ways eclipsed traditional treatment of illness and health maintenance. In response, efforts made by na kāhuna (Hawaiian medical practitioners) to restore the health of Hawaiians, combining both Native and introduced knowledge and practices, illustrate the determination of the people to maintain the value of their own knowledge and well-being. This chapter will briefly explore events and processes in Hawaiian history by outlining a political economy of health for the era that has contributed to an understanding that health is integral to the crafting of cultural and national identity.

Ali'i, Social Structure, and Transformation

Although physical health is the primary focus of medicine, we must not forget the larger social contexts that produce poor health. The physical health of Hawaiians is often linked to inequalities produced by colonial encounters that disparaged their beliefs, undermined their spiritual health and the knowledge of na kāhuna, and the alienation of Kanaka Maoli from the land. This is not to say that there was no hierarchy in the Hawaiian Islands before the arrival of Captain Cook in 1778. Hawai'i had one of the most hierarchical social systems in the Pacific. Described as similar to a feudal system, the basic classes of people included the ali'i nui (a chief of an island) who held the greatest amount of power, the kāhuna were the priestly class who served and enforced the dictates of the four main gods; Ku, Kane, Lono, and Kanaloa, the konohiki (headmen under the chief) and maka'āinana (the commoners, literal translation: people who looked to the land). This system was often amenable to merchants and traders who arrived in the Islands after Cook (Fuchs 1961; Howe 1996 [1988]). Merchants found Ali'i with whom they could negotiate trade agreements and the Ali'i had laborers, the maka'āinana, who could obtain natural resources from the land, such as sandal-wood. Merchants were also used by the Ali'i for their own political purposes. It is argued that Kamehameha I's skill at military tactics and the guns he acquired from traders were key factors in uniting the archipelago under one ruler.

The Ali'i were active agents in colonial encounters and the instigators of some of the major transformations in Hawaiian society. Some of their acts included cre-ating agreements between merchant traders and foreign governments, and abol-ishing long-held kapu (taboo). Scholars have discussed the motivations behind the actions of the Ali'i from the breaking of the 'ai kapu (the taboo against men and women eating food together) to the inclusion of foreigners as advisors in their uppermost political cabinets (Kame'eleihiwa 1992; Howe 1996 [1988]; Silva 2004). For example, after the death of Kamehameha I in 1819, Ka'ahumanu, Kamehameha II (Liholiho), the wife and son of Kamehameha I, and Keōpūolani (Liholiho's mother) decided to sit together and eat in public. In this one public act, the 'ai kapu would no longer be followed, paving the way for the dismissal of other kapu and religious rituals as well. One of the consequences of breaking the 'ai kapu and other rituals was that the kāhuna no longer held control over spiritual matters and over the daily tasks necessary to serve the will of the gods (Shiva 2004). These tasks were primarily performed by the maka'āinana. The transforma-tion of the kapu freed the maka'āinana from spiritual duties, but also gave them more time to work for the Ali'i (Kame'eleihiwa 1992). This dismantling of the religious structure through the breaking of the kapu, however, did not extend into the structure and practices of the medical kāhuna. As will be discussed later, the silencing of Hawaiian medical practices was accomplished through the outcries of the missionaries and some of their own medical practitioners. Shortly after the death of Kamehameha I and the shift in the kapu system, the first missionar-ies from the American Board of Commissioners for Foreign Missions arrived in 1820. Their disdain for the apparent "barbarism" of Hawaiians has been well documented in the memoir of Hiram Bingham (1847). The missionaries' ongoing dialogues with the Ali'i, while always tentative, also resulted in Ka'ahumanu being one of the first Hawaiians to publicly proclaim her conversion to Christianity.

Social hierarchy in Hawai'i at the time of early colonial encounters was in some ways amenable to the values of capitalism. Given the racial biases and desire for property exhibited by missionaries and merchant capitalists (categories that are not mutually exclusive) the locus of political power would not reside with the Hawaiian monarchy and the Ali'i for long. In the end, through the appropriation of land, waves of epidemics, and new forms of government intervention (such as registering ownership of land, licensing of physicians, and documentation of heritage/blood quantum), we find the ali'i disenfranchised and subject to the same stature as the maka'ainana. Thus, if we think of social inequality in terms of access to resources and in the way individuals are valued in society as factors in poor health, we begin to see the combined effects of colonization, missionization, and their toll on all Kanaka Maoli. The interaction of these social processes on discourses of health and the body will be explored further in this chapter. Given the multiple levels at which Hawaiian ideals were denigrated, regardless of hierarchies among Hawaiians themselves, what is important today for their survival and their national and cultural understanding of who they are is their emphasis on the relationship between land and health.

Alienation from the Land

One of the most damaging blows to the Hawaiians was the Māhele (division) in 1848. The Māhele was a transformation from the traditional communal land tenure system to private ownership. As American missionaries and businessmen required more acreage for their coffee, sugar, and pineapple plantations, and as they gained greater prominence as counselors in the monarchy there was a significant amount of economic and political power to push for a privatization of the land. Prior to the Māhele all the groups, the ali'i, konohiki, and the maka'ainana, cooperated with one another to subsist on the land. The land was divided by the ahupua'a system, a pie-shaped division from the mountains to the ocean. Segmenting the land in this way allowed the maka'ainana to share their food with the surrounding areas, giving the food to the ali'i and konohiki, who would in turn redistribute the food. This redistribution ensured that everyone had access to a variety of foods and maintained pono (balance or unity) with the land, the people, and the gods. The communal land tenure system was organized such that it could provide for all the people. It emphasized sharing and easy access to the land, while in the post-Māhele era private ownership emphasized restricted, unavailable land. The Māhele divided the land into the ali'i or crown lands, chiefs' lands, and the maka'āinana land or common land. Hawaiians, who emphasized sharing as part of their cultural identity, were unfamiliar with the foreigners' grab for private wealth and were at a disadvantage in a capitalist system (Kame'eleihiwa 1992). Kame'eleihiwa (1992) argues that when the Ali'i agreed to the Māhele, they believed that they were sharing the land or 'Āina[3] with the people and did not know that they were creating private ownership. This is based on two issues, one being that the word *māhele* also means to share; the second issue is that the 'Āina could only be owned by the gods, the akua, and the 'Āina was in essence an akua. Therefore no one could own an akua and thus no one could own the land. Because of the Māhele, Native Hawaiians had to present a claim to the Land Commission[4] before the individual could be awarded any land. According to Kame'eleihiwa, an appallingly small number (approximately 13 percent) of the Hawaiian population made claims to the Land Commission for their plot of land. Thus, many Hawaiians lost access to and control of the land that had sustained them and their ancestors for generations. It is notable that the Māhele took place after many had lost their lives to earlier epidemics of smallpox and syphilis, and during the same year (1848) as the flu, measles, and whooping cough epidemics that continued to take more lives. As a result, there were fewer individuals to make land claims, leaving much of the land available for purchase by foreigners. As Trask (1993) states with regard to the American missionaries and businessmen: "they came to do good, and did very well." Kame'eleihiwa notes that the disjuncture between the Hawaiian way of caring for and living off the land and the new capitalist way of using the land to make a profit not only led to a loss of physical access to the land but also to a loss of pono, that is, a loss of spirit and health.

The importance of Native Hawaiian attitudes towards the land is evident in many contemporary statements that have been carried down through history. For example, Hawai'i's state motto is a quote from Kamehameha IV, "Ua mau ke ea o ka 'Āina I ka pono," which has been translated as "The life of the Land is perpetuated by righteousness." This statement was made after the restoration of the Hawaiian kingdom following a British commander's failed attempt to acquire control of the land (Silva 2004). Kamehameha announced to the people in 1843 that the kingdom had a verbal agreement from the United States recognizing its independence. Furthermore, Great Britain and France had signed a joint resolution recognizing Hawai'i as an independent nation because it was "just and good." This phrase became the motto for the kingdom and ultimately the state motto. Yet, Native Hawaiians and researchers have argued that a more appropriate translation of the motto revolves around the word *ea*, which means both life and sovereignty (Kame'eleihiwa 1992, 1994; Trask 1993). Thus, the underlying meaning is, "The sovereignty of the land is perpetuated by pono, or by righteous behavior

(Kameʻeleihiwa 1994:36)." Silva (2004) has also researched the phrase focusing on the multiple meanings of the word pono. It is not only that pono can mean justice or righteousness, but that foreigners who sought to control the land interpreted it in terms of the righteousness associated with their belief in a Christian God. In contrast, for Kanaka Maoli it means a recognition that the perpetuation of justice is in the sovereignty of the land that is genealogically linked to the moʻi, aliʻi and people themselves. As Kameʻeleihiwa states, "For our Hawaiian ancestors, being an independent Nation, not being controlled by foreigners of any sort, was the very foundation of life. It was the life of the ʻaina, the land, the life of the aliʻi nui, the high chiefs, and the life of the makaʻāinana, the commoners" (1994:36).

Concerns about the poor health of Native Hawaiians initiated early attempts to return Hawaiians to the land. The ʻAhuahui Puʻuhonua O Na Hawaiʻi, organized in 1914 by a group of Hawaiians, encouraged people to purchase land and take care of the health of their family (McGregor 1989; Hasager 1994). As discussed by Hasager (1994), the group promoted change among the Hawaiians by drafting a "rehabilitation solution" that consisted of "living the traditional ʻHawaiian fish-and-poi' way, which indicates a way of life based on cultivating the taro gardens and fishing (1994:168)." The Hawaiian Homes Commission Act was the result of the organization's "rehabilitation solution." Its main goal was to return Hawaiians to the land of their ancestors. Unfortunately, the Act benefited a small number of people who actually obtained plots of land. The majority of land requests to the Hawaiian Homes Commission resulted in long waiting lists, with many Hawaiians dying before any award would ever be made. This is a situation that continues into the present. Many of the people I spoke with testified to the despair and anger they feel over watching their parents wait for land and are now waiting themselves. Importantly, according to Hasager (1994), the land that was set aside for the Hawaiian Homes Commission had already been rejected by capitalist entrepreneurs as unsuitable for farming. Lack of irrigation and poor soil content made living off the land extremely difficult. Hawaiians' inability to have access to the land of their ancestors, to fertile land for subsistence, further contributed to the decline in their health.

Foreigners' beliefs and business interests not only conflicted with Native Hawaiians' subsistence, their interests were also in opposition to spiritual attachments to the land. The concept of malama ʻaina is derived from the Kumulipo, the Hawaiian origin story. The Kumulipo also highlights the importance of the relationship between land and health. One version of the origin chant tells of Papa (earth mother) and Wākea (sky father) creating the Hawaiian Islands.

ʻO Wākea Kahikoluamea e a,   Wākea the son of Kahikoluamea,

ʻO Papa, Papa-nui-hānau-moku   Papa, Papa-nui-hānau-moku the

ka wahine;	wife;
Hānau Kahiki-kū, Kahiki-moe,	Kahiki-kū, Kahiki-moe, were born
Hānau ke 'āpapanu'u,	The upper stratum was born,
Hānau ke 'āpapalani,	The uppermost stratum was born,
Hānau Hawai'i, i ka moku	Hawai'i was born, the first-born of
makahiapo,	the islands,
Ke keiki makahiapo a laua . . .	The first-born of the two . . .
(Kamakau 1991:126)	

From the union of Wākea and Ho'ohōkūkalani (Papa and Wākea's daughter), a half-formed child named Hāloa-naka was born. The child was buried at the end of a house and there grew the first kalo/taro plant. Wākea and Ho'ohōkūkalani also gave birth to a second son, Hāloa, who is regarded as the ancestor of all Hawaiians (Kame'eleihiwa 1992). Since the kalo is considered the elder sibling of all Native Hawaiians, it is held in high esteem. From this creation story derives the responsibility Hawaiians have to take care of the land that feeds them and gives them life.

Alienation from the land resulted in both spiritual and physical death for Hawaiians. It signifies the consistent push of colonists to disenfranchise Natives from their land, leading to a political economy wherein options for all Native Hawaiians are constrained. Establishing the history of the seizure of Hawaiian land has become an important part of the process of re-territorializing the boundaries of Hawai'i and reestablishing the health of Native Hawaiians through their relationship to the land. Native Hawaiian symbols of land and history co-produce a salient image of a cultural identity that is embedded in narratives of health. By calling attention to the cultural and political dimensions of land, ancestors, and health, discourses of "natural" failures or biological "deficiencies" are questioned and the exercise of power is denaturalized.

Depopulation

As is the case for many native populations in the Americas and the Pacific, much of the loss of culture, land, and political power in the Hawaiian Islands is underpinned by the depopulation of the native people. Discourses of depopulation often focus on facets of population size, location/carrying capacity, and the health and morals of the indigenous people, with an implicit emphasis on configuring a context in which the population was either very small, not occupying the colonized territory, or well on its way to extinction because of supposedly uncivilized practices (Kirkby 1984; Thomas 1990; Anderson 2006). It has long been argued that the various discourses of depopulation typically convey a sense of inevitability that colonizers use to dismiss the indigenous populations' existence and claim political and economic rule of the territory for themselves (Maunier 1949; Wolf 1982; Kirkby 1984; Blaut 1993). For example, depopulation in Tasmania consisted of the violent and forcible removal of the aboriginal population from the land with the justification that they were not using the territory that the colonizers needed for their own homes and subsistence (Flood 2006). The depopulation of Tasmanian aboriginals from the land has been so complete that contemporary discourses of aboriginals center on Australia, forgetting the indigenous people of Tasmania and the Torres Straits; it is as if they were never there. In other cases, existing cultural practices were identified as already contributing to depopulation independent from the colonizers' presence. Locales such as Fiji (Thomas 1990) and the Philippines (Anderson 2006) were marked by discourses of depopulation that suggest that lack of hygiene, immoral practices, and "heathen" practices were the cause of the increasing demise of the native people. In Fiji, "polygamy," "fishing by child-bearing women," and "domestic dirt" were among some of the practices noted by colonists as the cause of increased native deaths (Thomas 1990:154–155). These a priori assumptions of demise further justified policies that served to "civilize" the indigenous population and included using local political structures to do so. As Thomas describes, incorporating chiefs as sources of information (such as asking them to record births and deaths) came with the intent of transforming practices that would result in mechanisms that affect a Foucauldian type of government that could be used to define and manage the population. What we must remember is that the knowledges and practices advocated by the colonizers set the framework for capitalist modes of production (Kirkby 1984). Drawing on Maunier (1949), Kirkby argues that "colonization is a capitalist achievement . . . an exercise of power which involves the emigration of people, capital and government, and that the exploration of a colony aims at economic profit as well as the subjection of the original inhabitants." Viewed in this way, discourses of depopulation are not only about identifying the deficiencies and absences within an indigenous culture thereby justifying the complete or partial passing of territory from the hands of one group to another, but rather offer insights on the effects of power and its internal workings on the lived experiences of the dispossessed. The contention over Kanaka Maoli dispossession and depopulation, and the silencing of their practices reflects the political dynamics that shift the blame from the colonial policies and social structure to the individual population and biological deficiencies, thus allowing colonial discourses of depopulation to appear natural and inevitable. Yet, when we examine the stories surrounding depopulation we find a political economy of health that is contested; indeed, it is fraught with debates over accurate information about health.

Almost any account of European contact with the Hawaiians begins with the overwhelming loss of life among the islanders. At first, many lives were lost to gonorrhea, syphilis, and tuberculosis; later, influenza and smallpox also took their toll on the Hawaiian population. Some accounts document the explorers' surprise at the speed with which sexually transmitted diseases spread from one island to another (Bushnell 1993). Other accounts testify to the captain's and crew's knowledge that the diseases they harbored in their bodies would wreak havoc on the native population, and their blatant disregard of that outcome when they were given permission to go ashore. For example, Stannard (1989) begins his book *Before the Horror* with the following passage:

> The injury these people receiv'd from us by communicating the certain destroyer of mankind [syphilis] is not to be repair'd by any method whatever . . . The man who has rob'd, murder'd and been guilty of all the catalogue of human crimes is innocent when compar'd to the one who did such a thing knowingly. (William Anderson, Captain Cook's Surgeon aboard *The Resolution*, commenting on the effects of their visit to Tonga in July 1777, 18 months before visiting Hawai'i and spreading the same disease to the Hawaiian people).

The possibility that Cook and his crew were aware of the ramifications of their actions speaks to the ways in which native populations were devalued even as they were first confronted. Captain Cook's arrival on the Hawaiian Islands and the diseases that followed will forever be linked to the depopulation of a once strong and healthy society.

According to Stannard (1989), Hawaiian depopulation is often overlooked or dismissed as insignificant. Part of this oversight has to do with the perceived degree of the depopulation. The Hawaiian Islands are small, and some have argued that there could not have been many islanders at the time of first contact. In fact, until recently most researchers had accepted estimates of between 200,000 and 400,000 Hawaiians prior to Cook's arrival (Fuchs 1961; Schmitt 1971).

Current research has challenged these numbers. Stannard (1989) estimates that there were actually between 800,000 and 1,000,000 pre-contact Hawaiians. One of Stannard's key contentions is that previous population estimates (made in 1778 by James King, a lieutenant on Cook's ship) were incomplete because they were based solely on the coastal population in Kealakekua Bay, on the lee-ward (dry) side of the island of Hawai'i. According to Stannard, people living in the fertile inland areas or the wet windward sides of the islands were not taken into account as King apparently assumed that the inland areas were unpopulated. Stannard argues that, given the technologies of the islanders, the carrying capacity of the Hawaiian Islands has been severely underestimated. Estimates have not taken into account the highly developed fishing and fish-pond techniques (aquaculture), the intensive agriculture that took place on many parts of the island, or the ahupua'a system (a system of sharing food among families that ranged from the ocean to the mountains). The amount of fertile land, and the sophisticated aquaculture and agriculture suggest that the carrying capacity of the islands was far more than originally estimated. Consider the fact that by 1878 there were only 48,000 Kanaka Maoli. Using Stannard's population estimate, hardly 100 years after Cook's arrival over 90 percent of the Hawaiian population was gone.

Stannard argues that both the lack of rigorous research into the size of the pre-contact population and the fact that the depopulation is rarely talked about in relation to the contemporary status of Hawaiians is the result of "historical amnesia" among Westerners. In order to establish an accurate history of the Hawaiian Islands, it is necessary, as Stannard notes, to continue to research and debate the size of the pre-contact population and depopulation. What is important about the debate over population estimates is the ability to lay claim to presumably unused land as well as to suggest that the number of deaths following the arrival of explorers and colonists was not very high. Even if we use a more conservative estimate of the population the decline associated with contact is still well over 50 percent.

A second issue relates to the effects of transformations in the social structure combined with the population's increased exposure to infectious diseases. An explanation that is most typically given for the demise of Natives is that they had no immunity to the diseases brought by foreigners. With the exception of tuberculosis, paleopathological research appears to support the contention that the other diseases (such as gonorrhea, syphilis, small pox and influenza) had yet to be introduced to the islands (Trembly 1997). The attribution of lack of immunity, however, should be more thoroughly questioned. First, the explanation of "lack of immunity" plays into a survival of the fittest and civilizing narrative (Martin 1995). A result of this thinking is support for a colonial contention that rule of the Hawaiian Islands by Euro-Americans was inevitable. Second, we must also think about how opportunistic infections take hold in humans whose immune systems are weakened through the effects of inequality (Wolf 1982; Farmer 1999).

The concept of a *syndemic* is one way to think about the social determinants of health and illness. Syndemic refers to the interaction of co-infections and social conditions that give rise to a greater burden of disease in some individuals and populations (Baer, Singer, and Susser 2003; Singer and Clair 2003). Thus, syndemics occur when individuals and groups are continually exposed to infectious diseases, when people live in environments where they do not have access to nutritious food, clean water, and housing, and are under persistent stress (Singer and Clair 2003).

These are all social contexts in which the immune system is compromised. The issue of co-infections arises because when the body is in the process of fighting or recovering from one infection, the compromised immune system is more susceptible to new infections. Consider the context in Hawai'i, within 60 years after the European encounter in 1798; first there was the exposure to sexually transmitted diseases and tuberculosis from the sailors, followed by a bubonic plague or cholera epidemic in 1804–1805, the flu, measles, and whooping cough in 1848, and smallpox in 1853. The picture painted here is not of a people unable to cope with encounters with foreigners; rather, it is a picture of a people whose health was compromised through rapid exposure to a multitude of infectious diseases, without a sufficient amount of time for their immune systems to recover.

The concept of a syndemic also demands that the effects of exposure to opportunistic infections be seen against the context of the social and structural stressors that Hawaiians were experiencing at the time. Scheder (2006) argues that we must account for potential psychoneuroimmunological (PNI) effects; in other words, PNI research focuses on the interaction between biology, cultural and individual meanings, and social inequality. Scheder calls our attention to the high death toll during the epidemics, alienation from the land, and the effects of colonization. Although she notes that there is insufficient paleopathological evidence to fully examine PNI effects, Scheder's argument moves us towards a more complete understanding of the depopulation of Hawaiians from their islands. For example, approximately 150,000 Hawaiians died in the 1804 cholera epidemic. Drawing on the work of Kemeny et al. (1994) that documents the effects of repeated bereavement on immune suppression (p. 43), Scheder argues that the grief among family and communities over the loss of so many loved ones may have created a significant amount of stress. Moreover, with the rapid death of so many individuals, ceremonial rituals related to caring for and burying loved ones were curtailed. Add to this the alienation of Hawaiians from their land as discussed in the previous section, and the denigration of Hawaiian ways by missionaries and colonizers that will be discussed later, an argument for a syndemic is far more compelling than a monocausal biological argument about lack of immunity resulting from a single infection.

Hawaiian Medicine as a Source of Self-determination and Denigration

While European-introduced diseases wreaked havoc on Native Hawaiians and the organization of their society, attacks were also being made on the ideological elements of Hawaiian health and medicine. The Europeans and Americans also brought to the Islands their medical practitioners, as well as their beliefs about the body and how it should be healed. Despite the fact that Western medicine was no more effective in dealing with the diseases of the time than Hawaiian medicine (Bushnell 1993), foreigners sought to impose Western medical beliefs and practices. Resistance to these views did occur, as evidenced by the licensing and organization of Hawaiian practitioners (Bushnell 1969, 1993), yet the attacks on the ideological system—kapu, and religious structure—that gave Hawaiian medicine its meaning led to a devaluation of its importance to Hawaiian life. The goal of the American and British immigrants and missionaries was the implicit colonization of Hawaiian minds through the complete transformation of their society and beliefs. More recently, this painful colonizing legacy has been reclaimed by Hawaiians and has become a point of resistance and a reminder of what was done and what must be overcome.

Among pre-contact Hawaiians, health was not just a matter of physical well-being, but also of spiritual and social well-being. The breaking of a kapu (taboo, prohibition), offending a spirit, or having an argument with a family member or friend weakened the mana, or life force found in people, animals, and objects. Weakened mana caused illness and disease, but it could be restored through the use of plants, animals, or anything in the natural environment, including the land, or through prayer to the gods or by restoring relationships with people who had been offended. The strong relationship between mind, body, and the social and natural environment meant that medical kāhuna treated both the spiritual and physical aspects of illness (Handy et al. 1934; Kamakau 1964; Bushnell 1993).

Medical kāhuna had an extensive knowledge of the body, the natural environment, and the Hawaiian gods. Although the quality of individual practitioners varied (as in any medical system) there were organized ways to train future kāhuna. As part of the priestly class, kāhuna were trained at heiau ho'ola (healing temples) as apprentices. These trainees were rigorously tested and supervised to ensure that they were making correct diagnoses and providing proper treatments. Kamakau (1964) lists several types of kāhuna lapa'au, from kāhuna ho'ohapai keiki who induced pregnancy and delivered babies, kāhuna haha who diagnosed by palpation, to kāhuna makani who treated the spirits of illness and kāhuna ho'opi'opi'o who used counteracting sorcery in their treatment (p. 98). If a kahuna wanted to specialize or learn a new type of healing he would seek out a heiau ho'ola with the kāhuna who specialized in that specific practice. Summoned by a member of the sick person's family, the kahuna would visit the sick person at home, diagnose the illness, and administer the appropriate treatments. Prayer, collection of specific plants, integration of family into the diagnosis and treatment, and strict diets were all part of the healing process. Thus, treating a sick person could take several days. The spiritual and physical well-being of pre-contact Hawaiians was not taken lightly. The importance of maintaining pono (balance or harmony) between the body, relationships with people, gods, and nature was evidenced in the medical practices of the kāhuna as part of the priestly class and in the formal organization of the system of treatment. As Bushnell notes in his work on the organization of pre-contact Hawaiian medical practices, kāhuna lapaʻau had to go through numerous steps in their training. They had to be trained at the appropriate heiau with well-known and respected kāhuna. Demonstration of their knowledge of the body, plants, spirits, and sorcery that could cause illness was imperative. Knowledge of all the ways of the god of the heiau at which they were trained was mandatory. Only kāhuna lapaʻau who had the established knowledge and educational pedigree through their heiau would be considered legitimate healers.

Post-contact transformations, such as the rise of the monarchy and the continued influx of colonizers and missionaries, set in motion a process of training and licensing that seemed more formal in the eyes of the foreigners. Despite the increased organization of kāhuna and their acceptance of some allopathic practitioners' knowledge, the kāhuna became the focus of the vilification of Hawaiian beliefs and practices by foreigners. Often, kāhuna were blamed for the continued deaths of Hawaiians from the waves of epidemics. As this July 1892 quote from *The Friend* (cited in Bushnell 1993:119) testifies:

> There is reason to believe that such murders constitute no small percentage of the causes of death that are swelling the immense mortality among Hawaiians. . . . The kahuna domination paralyzes the efforts of our skilled physicians to heal the people. The government employs physicians at great expense, but most of the people are prevented from obeying their prescriptions by the orders of the exorcisers to whose violent and destructive treatment they timidly submit. . . . The kahuna is the deadly enemy of Christianity and civilization. . . . They cannot think reasonably nor entertain sound opinions.

This quote suggests that the attack on medical kāhuna was intimately tied with the efforts of the Christian missionaries. Since the breaking of kapu in 1819 the role of the kāhuna had diminished. Because of the practical knowledge of the medical kāhuna, however, their importance in daily life was not severely affected. As such, they were viewed as a spiritual and practical threat to the "civilizing" efforts of the missionaries. Medical kāhuna mediated between the power of the gods, aliʻi (ruling class), and the practices of everyday life (Kameʻeleihiwa 1992; Buck 1993). Their ability to communicate with spirits and people bridged the boundaries between the worlds of the gods, aliʻi and commoners, reinforcing Hawaiian beliefs about illness and the actual practices used to deal with illness. Kāhuna practices in the everyday life of the makaʻāinana (commoner class) made them an integral part of the "ideological reproduction" of the Hawaiian social structure (Buck 1993). Yet, when Christian missionaries told the Natives that through conversion to Christianity they could attain everlasting life in the face of the epidemics, many Hawaiians turned away from the gods of their ancestors and the kāhuna lapaʻau in order to embrace Christianity and the promised life (Kameʻeleihiwa 1992). Given the strong connection between physical, spiritual, and psychological well-being, this attack on the kāhuna and their treatments was also a strong attack on the worldview of Native Hawaiians.

The move from Hawaiian knowledge and practices met with resistance from within the Hawaiian community. Malcolm Nāea Chun has translated Hawaiian-language newspapers from the 1800s, which has highlighted the concerted efforts that kāhuna made to save the lives of their people. As Chun's translation shows, one such effort to address the illness of the people by kāhuna was the 1867 Report of the ʻAhuahui Lā ʻau Lapaʻau of Wailuku, Maui, on Native Hawaiian Health. The ʻAhuahui Lāʻau Lapaʻau was a group of kāhuna organized to find solutions to the 1850s smallpox epidemic. Kamakau, a native Hawaiian historian in the 1800s, stated:

> In 1853, smallpox (maʻi puʻupuʻu hebera) came to Hawaii. This writer entered the houses and himself saw the many people who had been overcome by the destructive disease (maʻi luku), and the many dead. It was heartbreaking. . . . This writer is well acquainted with smallpox. He cured more than a hundred persons, and some are now alive because they were healed by his treatment in Kipahulu and Hana, because the government did not take care of those who got the sickness there. Kamakau (1964:105,106)

It was with this emergency in mind that the ʻAhuahui acted. The organization discussed four main questions:

> 1) Can only the Board of Health investigate and research medical treatments for the benefit of public health? Is it against the law for others to seek alternative treatments? 2) Are there appropriate Hawaiian medicines to treat diseases present throughout the Kingdom? 3) Is it possible using traditional medicinal treatments to diagnose and treat various diseases? and 4) Is it better to disregard traditional medicines and to rely on modern medicine [practiced] by the Board of health? (Chun 1994)

The President of the ʻAhahui, J.W.H. Kauwahi, believed that answering these questions would "provide the means to validate the traditional practitioners and to disbar those quacks [people who were not properly trained] from practicing." (Chun 1994:iv). The ʻAhahui interviewed kāhuna from all over the island of

Maui and compiled the interviews; these interviews are published in Hawaiian and English in Chun's book *Must We Wait in Despair* (1994). While it is not known whether the 'Ahahui ever presented its findings to the Board of Health, in 1868 the legislature established a Hawaiian Board of Health that licensed eligible kāhuna to practice Hawaiian medicine. Although the kāhuna were still despised by the white population, their practice was accepted as legal. In 1893 with the overthrow of the Hawaiian kingdom, the Hawaiian Board of Health was also abolished and was not reinstated until thirty years later.

It is clear from the goals of 'Ahahui that by this time foreign practitioners had full control over who would receive allopathic medicines, which were hard to find and expensive. In addition, the foreigners wished to control the use of Hawaiian medicines. The 'Ahahui was one effort by Native Hawaiians to stem the rising tide of colonization. This example is significant because it shows that Hawaiians did not just give up their practices for the more "civilized" ones of the foreigners. The publication of 'Ahahui's work shows the existence of concerted Hawaiian efforts to resist colonization of their minds and bodies.[5]

Contemporary Native Hawaiian Health

At a time when many were inspired by the civil rights' and feminist movements, young Hawaiians also began to contest the history they learned in schools and textbooks and began instead to focus on the stories told to them by their parents and grandparents (Trask 1993). Hawaiians organized to save sacred areas such as Kahoʻolawe, which is a small island (approximately 45 square miles) off the southwest side of Maui. This island was seized by the military in 1941 and subsequently used for bombing practice.[6] In the mid-1970s the organization, Protect Kahoʻolawe, worked to stop the destructive bombing of this land and to claim once again the right to mālama 'āina (care for the land). During this time there was also a push to resolve the dramatic health and "social problems" plaguing Native Hawaiian communities.

A report published by the Liliʻuokalani Trust Advisory Board in 1962 prompted studies of Hawaiian communities. This report stated that Hawaiians were overrepresented in essentially all categories of "social problems." Not only were Hawaiians overwhelmingly present in the "social problems" category, later studies also showed startling rates of chronic diseases as discussed earlier (Alu Like 1985; Office Technology Assessment 1987; Wegner 1989). The inability to access land and nutritious foods, the introduction of high-fat Western diets, with the addition of canned foods and fast food from outlets such as McDonald's and Jack in the Box, created a nutritional nightmare. Cigarettes and alcohol have also played significant roles in causing diseases and other social problems. Concerns about health and social problems have become rallying points in the discourse over Native Hawaiian identity.

In an effort to combat these health inequalities, the 1974 Congress passed the Native American Act, which provided funds to private and public agencies serving Native Americans, which included Native American Indians, Alaskan Natives, and Hawaiian Natives. Many of these funds were used for education, economic growth, and to address the health problems of Hawaiians. In 1988 the Federal government passed the Native Hawaiian Health Care Improvement Act (Public Law 100–579), which led to the creation of Papa Ola Lokahi, the coordinating agency, which works with five Native Hawaiian Health Care Systems. These agencies' tasks include promoting primary care services, implementing preventive services, and organizing and creating easy access to Native Hawaiian Health Professionals. In addition, studies of Native Hawaiian health have increased over the last 30 years, becoming a growing field of research for public health officials, anthropologists, physicians, psychologists, and others.

In the past many researchers focused on the Native Hawaiian belief that health is contingent upon the state of social relationships (e.g., Linnekin 1985; Shook 1986; Ito 1985, 1987, 1999). Health as a social relationship is based on the idea of maintaining pono (harmony or balance) in relationships. According to Ito, "the shameful exposure of a failure of the aloha ideal leaves one vulnerable to the retributive attacks of illness or misfortune by the object, the victim of such manini (stingy) or lili (jealous)" (1987:56). Although social relational health is an important part of a Native Hawaiian health framework, a focus on what I call land-based health has not been as evident in earlier scholarly research. Land-based health promotes a return to growing and eating traditional foods. At another level a return to working and eating from the land would also facilitate the improvement of spiritual and cultural health. The emphasis on land and its importance to personal and cultural health is crucial to the promotion of a Hawaiian cultural identity (e.g., Kame'eleihiwa 1992, 1994; Trask 1994). These are problems, however, that researchers at the forefront of Native Hawaiian health issues had not previously addressed.

There have been two successful programs that emphasize a return to the Native Hawaiian diet, both through eating traditional foods and by obtaining that food through aquaculture and gardening. Both these programs, the Wai'anae Diet Program (Shintani et al. 1991) and the Moloka'i Heart and Diet Study (Curb et al. 1991) have provided evidence that a return to the Native Hawaiian diet would indeed improve the health of Hawaiians.

Discussions of land-based health expand the focus on pono to include its essential connections to the land (Kame'eleihiwa 1992, 1994; Blaisdell and

Mokuau 1994; Gomes 1994). The Wai'anae diet promotes the belief that when Hawaiians maintain a healthy relationship with the land, the land, through food, healing medicine, and spirituality, will take care of Hawaiians:

> And when enough Hawaiians are lōkahi (one) within themselves . . . with the land through the food they eat . . . with all Hawaiians and the Papa and Wakea . . . then the health of the people will be restored, and the cultural strengthening of the Hawaiian people will follow. (Shintani and Hughes 1993)

According to a Native Hawaiian cultural model of health, however, Native Hawaiians must have access to Hawaiian land. The relative absence of health, when viewed from the land-based model, is entwined with the politics of land distribution in Hawai'i (e.g., Gomes 1994). A move back to a traditional Hawaiian diet becomes an embodiment of a rejection of foreign foods and ways. The adoption of a Wai'anae diet challenges people to reclaim a past in which Native Hawaiians are viewed as a healthy, active, and independent people; this is an act against the syndemics that have plagued the people since contact. A movement towards that state is not only a psychological step, but is also a call to action, marking a change in behavior and a revitalization of Hawaiian identity.

Remembering the ancestors' past and charting positive directions for the future extends to health promotion in local clinics and for Native Hawaiian practitioners. Even a cursory scan of health-related brochures targeted toward Native Hawaiians reveals the use of culturally significant designs and symbols to represent the organization. Typically a logo for a health organization will have at least one of three specific symbols woven into its design: the image of a kupuna (an elder), which always evokes respect; the island that the organization is serving, symbolizing the land base that provides health; and the kalo plant, a local food source and more importantly the elder brother as described in the Kumulipo (origin story). The logo of Hui No Ke Ola Pono a Native Hawaiian health center on Maui, contains a kalo plant in the center of the picture, the ti leaf lei surrounding the kalo and a medicine bowl (Figure 1.1). It is important to note that the ti leaf lei is placed in the shape of the island Maui, representing the importance of the island and the land base. Moreover, the ti leaf lei is sometimes worn by kāhuna and physicians as a way to ward off evil and summon good. Thus, the ti leaf lei surrounding Maui can be thought of as warding off elements that may cause poor health and calling in good health.

Likewise, in a brochure for a seminar on Hawaiian healing methods sponsored by Ho'ola 'o LomiLomi Lapa'au Clinic a pair of hands holding a kalo plant is the primary logo. On the brochure, beneath the kalo are the words "Our Heritage," which are placed beside a kahuna, who is a specialist, priest

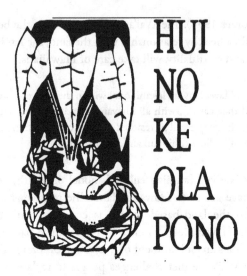

Figure 1.1. Logo for Hui No Ke Ola Pono, Maui Native Hawaiian Health Organization. Courtesy of Hui No Ke Ola Pono, www.huinomaui.org

or healer, typically an elder, a kupuna. The elder holds in his arms a bundle of awa (also known as kava, this plant promotes relaxation and relief of muscle pain). These images and the words "our Heritage" evoke links to the ancestors. The cover of the Wai'anae book of health also shows and image of young Hawaiian with a kalo plant, root and leaves behind person. These key symbols have gained widespread use in the current struggle by Native Hawaiians to reclaim their history and revitalize their cultural identity. That these symbols are used to signify health tells us that Native Hawaiian health involves more than merely attending to the physical body; it is intimately tied to a communion with ancestors (kūpuna), with the land and kalo that they care for and that in turn cares for them. These symbolic relationships reflect a tethering of people to the land through their caring for, consumption of, and ultimate return to it. The kalo stalk is called the hā, which also means the number four, a breath or life. The 'ohā refers to the off shoots of kalo representing the future generations or the children of the kalo. 'Ohā is also the root of the word 'ohana, or family. Although both kalo leaves and roots are used for subsistence, and the stalk is used to propagate new plants, we are often provided with an image of the whole plant. Showing the whole plant suggests the importance of remaining rooted in the land from which the family will grow, producing more food and people. The whole plant may also suggest the importance of pono, that is, of harmony with parts of life and family as part of health and healing. The use of kalo as a symbol on health advertisements is not simply an indicator of eating healthy foods, it is a statement of the political and cultural link between land, kalo, ancestors, and a potential for Native Hawaiian health.

Kāhea ola (the call to life), a phrase used in the Wai'anae Comprehensive Health Organization (Shintani and Hughes 1993), is more than a call to restore the health of the physical body. It is a call to the Hawaiian people, to the meaning and symbols of their culture, to the land, to fully restore that which has been waiting, dominated by Western ideologies. The themes of history, land, and health, as shown through the logo designs, are intertwined, working together to illuminate the politics of health and to redefine Native Hawaiian culture and identity.

Health as a Marker of Hawaiian Cultural Identity and the Imagined Community

King (1987) has noted that it is only by addressing the denigration of Native Hawaiian culture by foreigners that a decolonization of the mind can begin, which will result in a restoration of health. Decolonization of the mind is integral to the restoration of health, and necessarily includes an understanding of Hawaiian history. The health practices of Native Hawaiian ancestors, the negative impact of European and American contact, the transformation of Hawaiian medicine as a site of denigration and resistance, and the state of Native Hawaiians' current health are all facets of the political economy of health and major elements in the construction of shared cultural and individual identity.

Increased exposure to Native Hawaiian beliefs about health has taken place in a politicized era, not only in terms of a growing sovereignty movement but also with increasing calls for Congressional funding for research. It is more often than not the case that issues of health and life are intimately tied to ideology and politics. I would caution, however, against writing off the importance of the links between history, health, and land as an "invention of tradition" or ethnopolitics. The relative importance of these issues has changed over the years, not because life and death did not matter to the Hawaiian population, but rather because the life and death of Native Hawaiians was not deemed an important matter by the dominant society.

Native Hawaiians share a complex and painful past: historical events such as the mass depopulation of their ancestors from the islands, the legacy of contact with outsiders that denigrated and erased traditional Hawaiian ways and values, and the current poor economic and health status of Hawaiians deeply affect Native Hawaiian identity. The subsequent chapters will elaborate on how Native Hawaiians look to the past for answers about who they are and how they should act. The responses to these questions work towards building a collective memory, an imagined community, and a healthy body, but more importantly represent recognition of the politics of health and a *preferred* Native Hawaiian way to build identity and deal with the problems of today.

Endnotes

1. Historical information in this chapter has been summarized from Bushnell (1993), Kamakau (1991), Kame'eleihiwa (1992), and Malo (1951).
2. While Hawai'i is certainly west of the United States, to talk about the West is also to talk about the hegemonizing ideologies associated with the United States. When referring to the United States and ideologies associated with the United States many of my interviewees used the term the "West."
3. Kame'eleihiwa argues that Āina should be capitalized as it is the bodily form of a god.
4. The Land Commission was a board of five individuals, primarily U.S. missionaries and businessmen, appointed by Kamehameha III in 1845 to organize and rule on land claims.
5. Silva's 2004 research of Hawaiian-language newspapers during this same era is a remarkable analysis of Native Hawaiian resistance to colonial domination.
6. See Aluli and McGregor (1994) for information on the protection and restoration of Kaho'olawe.

2

MANAGING IDENTITY, CONTEXT, AND METHODS

Conducting a cultural study in a place that has been heavily dominated by colonial, missionary, and tourist influences is a questionable endeavor in the opinion of many people, both lay and academic. One aspect of that questioning came in the form of joking that began the moment I finally decided to conduct my field research in the Hawaiian Islands. Friends, family, and colleagues made comments such as "*Sure* you're going there to work?" "It must be nice to interview at the beach," or "Getting paid to work on your tan," accompanied by little chuckles and knowing smirks. These comments, while seemingly innocent and all in good fun, reflect a romanticized vision of the Hawaiian Islands as a place of leisure and relaxation. Although actually "working" in Hawai'i was not an issue among academics, studying a population that might not even have a "Hawaiian" culture anymore was problematic. It was suggested that the Hawaiians had been so severely depopulated and "Westernized" that they no longer had a culture[1] of their own. In other words, because the sociopolitical structure or daily practices were not as they were prior to contact there would be little of the "other" to study. The "romanticized" and "lost culture" perspectives of Native Hawaiians are seemingly opposite sides of the same coin. Hawai'i holds both the stigma of being a place for the consumer, the foreign tourist who is there for a leisurely vacation (a vacation, in part, from the demands of Western culture) and a place that has so physically and culturally succumbed to and been commodified by Western hegemony that it has no "real" culture left to study.

Hawai'i's incorporation into the global arena, not just as an economically assimilated site but a politically absorbed one as well, has obviously raised some questions about the existence of Hawaiian culture and even about the dimensions of the culture that has supposedly been lost. Despite the view of Hawaiian culture as static before Western contact, as with all societies, change has been continual for the inhabitants of the Hawaiian Islands. The original inhabitants arrived around AD 200 and were later joined and further transformed by migrants from the Society Islands. Over the span of approximately 1500 years, Hawaiians experienced many changes in their way of life, social structure, and religion. Hawaiians developed complex systems of agriculture and aquaculture, and a means to redistribute resources so that no one went hungry (Chapter 1). Hawai'i also had one of the most highly stratified social systems in the Pacific. There were small chiefdoms and districts on each island, and a complex religion with many gods and kapu (a system of prohibitions and sacred objects and people). The encroachment of Europeans and Americans on the islands, however, was staggering. Over the course of 150 years, all the islands were unified under one Hawaiian king, over 90 percent of the population died, work changed from subsistence to the export of natural resources, the kapu system was abolished, Christianity became the predominant religion, the communal land tenure system was dramatically transformed to private property, the monarchy was overthrown by American businessmen, and the islands were annexed by the United States and ultimately made the fiftieth state.

Given these significant transformations of Hawaiian culture and society, the argument that Hawai'i is not a valid place to conduct a study can be viewed not only as situating culture and identity as static, fixed, and immutable, but also as part of a colonial discourse that erases island history, colonial domination, and self-determination in the Islands. Hawai'i is not the only example where this erasure of history has occurred. Indeed, the bikini bathing suit, designed by Louis Reard and unveiled in 1946, just four days after the first atom bomb test on Bikini atoll, is a prime example of the erasure of colonial history through commodification. In discussing the relationship between the forced displacement of the Bikini Islanders,[2] so that their islands could be used as a nuclear test site, and the expected excitement over the atom-sized swim suit, Teaiwa (1994) has argued that:

> The sacrifice of Islanders and military personnel during nuclear testing in the Pacific cannot be represented without threatening the legitimacy of colonial power, so nuclear technology becomes gendered and domesticated. In the end the female body is appropriated by a colonial discourse to successfully disguise the horror of the bomb (1994:92).

Focusing on the sexualized image of a female in a bikini shifts our attention away from the continued displacement of the Bikinians and nuclear destruction that took place on their islands. Similar to the discourses of depopulation, the U.S. government felt the removal of the population in 1946 (approx. 167 people living on Bikini atoll) was so small that few people would be affected. Today, there are an estimated 4200 Bikinians who cannot live on the atoll because of the lethal radiation pollution from the bombing. And yet when we hear the word "bikini" we think of the bathing suit and not the bomb (Teaiwa 1994), an image that is perpetuated by the image of Rita Hayworth painted on the bomb and naming it "Gilda" (Caputi 1991). Thus, the bikini-clad female "bombshell" was used to erase the horrors of the metal-clad atom "bomb."

An examination of the mechanisms used to commodify Hawai'i suggests a similar process of erasure. Buck's 1993 study of the history of hula has shown how the hula performed for tourists ultimately erases the history of the once-sovereign nation and the subsequent overthrow of the monarchy in the minds of the larger population. Hula's strong tie to the remembrance of Native Hawaiian ancestors and its use as a capitalist commodity in tourism constructs it as one of the most valued and contested bodily practices (e.g., Buck 1993; Trask 1993; Stillman 2001; Silva 2004).[3] Through the mele (song or chant) and movement of the dancer, knowledgeable viewers are reminded of Hawaiian genealogies (of kings and gods alike), meanings of place, and the history of the ancestors. The movement of the body in hula, however, was viewed as obscene by the early missionaries in Hawai'i. At a time when foreigners were exercising power in numerous professions, from counseling, to the monarchy, and the island newspaper business, much was made of the "lascivious" hula movements (Stillman 1998; Silva 2004). The missionaries' disdain for hula and their lack of cultural or historical understanding of it ultimately led to the dance form being outlawed.

Decades after the outlawing of hula and other practices such as he'e nalu (surfing), King Kālakaua (the second to last monarch) brought these practices back into the public sphere. Indeed, hula was publicly performed at his coronation in 1874. Silva's 2004 superb book *Aloha Betrayed* documents Kālakaua's dedication to "preserving and perpetuating" Hawaiian culture. This goal was accomplished, in part, by providing opportunities for Kanaka Maoli to read their own history in the Hawaiian newspapers where Kālakaua published mo'olelo (stories), chants, genealogies, and the Kumulipo (Silva 2004).[4] The sharing of history in print form reminded the people of their heritage. Reviving hula was another mechanism through which history was preserved and perpetuated. With the history written and in place, hula once again became a practice that was used to retell Hawaiian history and legitimize Hawaiian knowledge through the body (Silva 2004). In the present milieu this embodied history, however, is also a representation of capitalist production. The soft, seductive body of the hula dancer is productive not only because it is controlled and self-disciplined through practice, but also because it is a *product* for tourist consumption.

Hula, as it is performed in the many hotels and nightclubs across the Hawaiian Islands, is also gendered, presenting the female body as an object to be consumed. As tourists gaze at the graceful female bodies, however, they are not reminded of Hawaiian history; rather, they are lulled into the relaxing sounds of the island paradise (Buck 1993; Trask 1993). These performances ignore the depopulation of the islands, struggles over conversion to Christianity, the overthrow of the monarchy, immigration of other populations, and the continued political and economic domination of the islands through tourism and capitalism. The persistence of hula in the commodified sphere of tourism is presented as if these political struggles never happened. The presentation of bodies that can be consumed, such as the exotic Pacific beauty in the "little grass skirt" or in a skimpy bikini, for the foreign tourist obscure the historical domination that Island nations have endured. As Teaiwa noted, "the emptiness of commodity consumption is only benign if we ignore the malign effects of the bikini's co-commodity, the bomb (1994:95)." Claiming that there is no culture left to study or that Hawai'i is merely a place for leisure is clearly linked to a colonial discourse that is disguised in a veil of consumerism.

Despite the intersection of representations of Hawai'i as a capitalist paradise made for the tourist or as a lost culture, Native Hawaiians have refused to allow their history to be obscured. For instance, the rise of Punana Leo (Hawaiian-language immersion schools), voyages of the vessel Hokule'a, traditional healing methods, and restoration of kalo gardens and fish ponds were often cited to me as examples of current efforts to revitalize Hawaiian knowledge. The institutionalization of Hawaiian language immersion schools is a significant achievement. In 1983 a group of Hawaiian language teachers formed the grassroots organization Aha Punana Leo, Inc., The Nest of Voices Corporation (Aha Punana Leo, Inc. 1998). Beliefs about the demise of the Hawaiian language and laws that prohibited teaching Hawaiian in schools were only a few of the obstacles that the organization faced. Teaching Hawaiian in schools had been outlawed when English was made the official language in 1896. What began as a small Punana Leo preschool in Kekaha, Kaua'i, funded only by tuition and parent help, grew to nine schools across the islands and led to the overturning of laws prohibiting the teaching and funding of the Hawaiian language in primary, middle, and high schools. In 2002 the first Masters' thesis completely written in Hawaiian was accepted at the University of Hawai'i in Hilo. The reemergence of the Hawaiian language serves as a symbol of survival on the islands and as a means to "decolonize the minds" of Hawaiians.

The building and sailing of the Hokuleʻa was another significant event in the Hawaiian renaissance. The Hokuleʻa, a double outrigger canoe, was built as an experiment by the Polynesian Voyaging Society to show the sailing character-istics of the craft design, and as Finney (1978) argues, the existence of the craft has put to rest debates that suggested that the Polynesian claims of ancestors navigating from Kahiki (thought to be Tahiti) were mere myths (Finney 1977, 1978). In 1976 the crew of the Hokuleʻa crossed the Pacific Ocean from Hawaiʻi to Tahiti by using the stars, moon, sun, and ocean swells to navigate their course (see Lewis 1972 for more on these navigation skills). Since that time the Hokuleʻa has made return trips to Tahiti and to Aotearoa (New Zealand). In 1995 the Polynesian Voyaging Society built another craft, the Hawaiʻiloa. These two vessels are evidence of the sophistication of Hawaiian and Polynesian technology and knowledge, and of Hawaiian ancestry, the "roots" of Hawaiian culture (Finney 1977, 1978). Recently, Tengan (2008) has provided an ethnographic account of the organized efforts by men to remake their Native masculinity through Hale Mua (men's house). Over the course of my fieldwork, the people I worked and lived with used these achievements to make it clear that their culture and iden-tity as Native Hawaiians would not be erased. For some of those I worked with, these symbols and practices were part of their active engagement with Hawaiian knowledge and for others it was sufficient to know what was available to them; in either case, however, the Hawaiian renaissance speaks to the larger issues of cultural resilience and change in the context of colonial and neocolonial domina-tion. The insistence on the value of Kanaka Maoli knowledge and the ability to practice that knowledge in the contemporary era are more than acts of resistance against colonial dominance, they are counter-hegemonic moves in that they place Native knowledge parallel to the dominant discourse and illuminate an alternate path that can be made available to contemporary Hawaiians.

Field Sites

There are several islands in the Hawaiian archipelago from which I could have conducted my study. During a preliminary trip I visited four of the more popu-lated islands; Oʻahu, Maui, Hawaiʻi, and Kauaʻi (see Figure 2.1). As when con-ducting most research, a key concern was finding a place to live. Although I had a couple of offers to live with families on other islands, I eventually choose to live and work on the islands of Maui and Hawaiʻi where I was accepted into the homes of two very generous families who made room for me even though they did not really have much space. In addition, the small towns they live in were appropriate for the research I wanted to conduct.

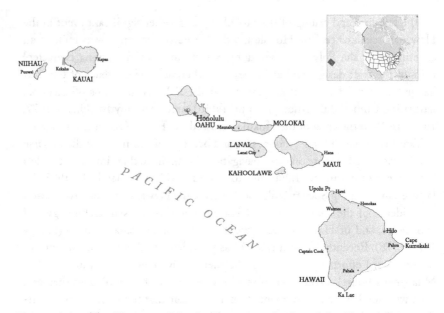

Figure 2.1. The Hawaiian Islands. The national atlas of the United States of America, U.S. Geological Survey, U.S. Department of the Interior, 2003, www. nationalatlas.gov [accessed August 4, 2009].

I was interested in talking with Native Hawaiians who live in small towns, who were somewhat dispersed throughout the community, and who had access to supermarkets, strip malls, clinics, and fast food. These criteria would also enhance the comparison with the Native Hawaiians I would talk with in Southern California, most of whom live in suburban areas. Even though off-islanders are dispersed throughout various communities in California, many find ways, through civics clubs and other events, to socialize with other Native Hawaiians.

The town of Hana, on the island of Maui, exemplifies my reasons for not wanting to study a small, close-knit Native Hawaiian community. For most people on Maui, Hana is a very special place. This beautiful rural area with its fauna and waterfalls is hard to get to and, to a certain extent, is secluded. Many people who live in the Hana district, which includes the small village of Keane (where Linnekin 1985 conducted her research), still farm kalo and are said to constitute a very intimate and closed community. In the minds of many Native Hawaiians with whom I spoke, Hana remains one of the last places where one can still live a truly Hawaiian lifestyle. Despite the fact that Hana has been a minor tourist destination since the 1970s and most of the population is employed by the local hotel, I was told that people in Hana still farmed the land, fished, and maintained all the close family networks that are necessary to a "traditional" Hawaiian life. I was told that because Hana is relatively secluded people who lived there did not have to deal with continuous interference from the outside. Only on Maui did the people I spoke with draw on the Hana lifestyle for good or bad as a comparison for Hawaiian living. This idealized Hawaiian community does not fit the life situations of most Native Hawaiians. I wanted to see how people who do not have the opportunity to live in such a "secluded" area, and had many opportunities for farming and engaging in rural Hawaiian practices, come up with strategies for dealing with their health dilemmas in what they would consider a Hawaiian way.

Fieldwork for this study took place in three different locations: Maui, Hawai'i, and southern California. The 2000 census estimates that there are 239,655 Native Hawaiians living on-island and approximately 161,507 living in the continental United States. These numbers represent a significant shift in the off-islander population, from 34 percent in the 1990 census to 40 percent of all Native Hawaiians counted in the 2000 census (Malone and Shoda-Sutherland 2005). Malone and Shoda-Sutherland have also found that Native Hawaiians living off-island are more likely to have a college degree, white collar jobs, and are less likely to live in poverty (12.4 vs. 16 percent), than on-islanders. Given the increasing numbers of Native Hawaiians living off-island, this approach illuminated the importance of the political economy and the intersections between cultural identity, health, land, and history within and between the people who assisted me with this research.

The Big Island

On the island of Hawai'i (more commonly known as the Big Island) I lived in Waimea, in the town of Kamuela. Located below the slopes of Mauna Kea, Kamuela rises 2,500 ft. above sea level, and is home to Parker Ranch (at the time, the third-largest ranch in the United States). At the time of this research, Kamuela has all the features of many small towns in the U.S. mainland, including a McDonalds in the main strip mall. In addition, Kamuela hosts a variety of cultural events, including the annual Aloha Festival's Paniolo Parade. The total population of the Big Island is 97,197, of whom only 23,120 are Hawaiians (19.2 percent). The total population of Kamuela is 9,052, of whom 2,197 (24 percent) are Hawaiian. Many of the Hawaiians I spoke with lived on or near Hawaiian Homes land (land allocated by the state on which only Native Hawaiians and their family may live and own property) in Kamuela. As a result of the networks I established in Kamuela, my interviews were conducted only on the West and

North half of the Big Island, ranging from the Kohala coast across the island to the city of Hilo. As is common in Hawai'i, most of the people I knew worked two or more jobs just to meet their financial obligations. They relied heavily on family networks for child care and other types of non-paid work to defray living costs.

Maui

Maui attracts an assortment of tourists, as well as spiritualists and other New Agers. Living in Maui was very different from life on the Big Island. I lived in the small town of Haiku (near Pa'ia), but most of my interviews took place in Wailuku and Lahaina. Wailuku is the main city in Maui, with the principal airport, a community college, a large shopping mall, many small strip malls, and several hospitals; Wailuku is similar to growing urban cities on the mainland.

Maui has a total population of 84,585 of whom 15,919 are Hawaiians (15.8 percent). Although, like Wailuku, having many urban amenities, Lahaina had many more hotels and was much more of a tourist city. Many of the people I spoke with in Lahaina worked for the local hotels.

Southern California

After the state of Hawai'i, California has the second largest population of Hawaiians. Of the 60,048 Native Hawaiians living in California, approximately 10 percent live in Orange County (2000 Census), which is where the majority of people I spoke with resided. Many of these Hawaiians maintain networks with other Hawaiians both in California and on the islands and continually travel "back home" to visit family and to attend a variety of Hawaiian cultural events, such as the Merrie Monarch Festival and Hula Competitions. Na Mamo, a Hawaiian club devoted to perpetuating Hawaiian culture in Southern California, hosts the annual E Hula Mau, which is hailed as the largest hula competition outside of the Islands. There has also been an increase in the offering of Hawaiian language courses by Hawaiian civics clubs, and greater attendance at many of the yearly cultural events, such as E Hula Mau, Ho'olaule'a, and Aloha Expo, to name a few.

From 1994 to 1996 I first lived on the island of Hawai'i, then Maui, and later completed my research at the final site in Southern California. Numerous observations, field notes, fortuitous conversations, and structured interviews comprise the data that I draw on. A total of 54 structured interviews with Native Hawaiians were completed.[5]

Of the structured interviews the mean age of the participants for both islands was 42.8 years. In Orange County, the mean age was 43 years. Despite the similarity in age for the three sites, there is a large disparity in income between on-islanders and off-islanders. The average household income was $20,615 for the on-islanders with whom I spoke. This low level of income is indicative of Native Hawaiians living on-island. Typically, as did most all of the participants, on-islanders occupy low-level, service-sector jobs. Most all the managerial, high-tech, teaching, and nursing jobs go to people imported from the mainland or to other immigrants; this fact, to many of my interviewees, is evidence of neo-colonial attitudes towards islanders. In contrast, off-islanders had an average household income of $60,750.[6] Although both Hawai'i and California have high costs of living, the difference in income levels reveals the constraints on opportunities for Native Hawaiians living on-island. In contrast to the importation of professionals to the islands, many of the off-islanders I spoke with migrated to the mainland to attend college or obtain access to better opportunities for professional work that were not available in Hawai'i. As will become apparent through the on-Islanders' and the off-Islanders' perceptions of health, the difference in income and education between the two groups influenced their narratives on the responsibility for health and health care.

Managing Identity: Looking Right, Behaving Right

Gaining entry into a Hawaiian community is not easy, as my experiences in the following section suggest. Even when a researcher knows where most of the Hawaiian population is living, one cannot simply knock at each door and ask to interview the head of the household. For me, gaining entry involved an extended period of rapport building. I had a few Native Hawaiian friends who could introduce me to people, and "vouch for my integrity." Behaviors play a large role in determining whether or not an individual is considered part of the community, and this line of thinking even extends into one's ability to meet individuals. I was told many times and by many people that Hawaiians watch for signs in your behavior, evaluating your conduct. Depending on what they observe, they will decide whether or not to talk to you.

Debates about representations of islands and island life inform, in part, our understanding of larger structural issues such as colonialism and inequality as well as giving rise to particular subjectivities, ways of seeing oneself in the world. Hawai'i for tourists is often viewed as familiar. Cleansed of colonial struggles, as suggested by the discussion of hula, it is represented as our island paradise. Moving beyond the familiarity created by tourism, however, I uncovered many ambiguities in representations of others and of my own identity. The ways in which I positioned myself vis-a-vis the academy and as a supporter of Hawaiian rights and the daughter of a man born and raised on the Islands[7] was very important. I took for granted the fact that my appearance engendered reactions that categorized me either as an accepted insider or a rejected outsider. I very much looked the part of a Hawaiian Islander, although I am not, and was not raised on-island. People I encountered, however, often mistook me for a Hawaiian or as someone who was raised on island. When I failed to meet their expectations, the disjuncture was immediately known. The incongruity between my behavior, in speech or action, and their expectation was visible not only by those observing me but also in my observations of their reaction, including the shock on the faces of those I was talking to, the uncomfortable moments of silence while I waited and watched their categorization, and the sense I had of being recategorized from insider to ambiguous subject.[8]

After reflecting on these incidents and on the observable transformation of my identity as reflected in other peoples' faces, I realized that anthropologists take for granted that we have little idea of how to behave culturally when we arrive at our field site. As anthropologists we are trained to understand that not only might the context around us be "unfamiliar," but our speech, mannerisms, and expectations of behaviors may be equally "unfamiliar" to the people with whom we live. In other words, we "know" that we do not know how to behave properly and we take for granted that the people we live with also "know" that we do not know how to behave. The increase in studies conducted by "natives" of their own communities, or by people who do not fit the stereotypical "white researcher," however, has complicated this assumption. At first glance we look like we belong, so those around us categorize us as belonging to their group and develop their expectations accordingly. Failure to meet those expectations, however, can become extremely disturbing; physical characteristics and behaviors do not coincide, and interaction becomes difficult because neither person is quite sure what to do next. In sum, managing identity was often out of my control. People I came into contact with noticed my brown skin, brown eyes, brown hair, and quiet personality and classified these as the symbols of someone who lives on island and decided what they expected of me: that I was not "strange" and that I fit in . . . or did I?

Even when one appears to fit in, the way in which one behaves among Native Hawaiians plays a big role in one's acceptance into the community. Nohea, who was born in Hawai'i and lived on the mainland for approximately 15 years, recently moved "home." She explained some of her experiences with her community as one who belonged, but also as one who is keenly aware of the differences from living on the mainland. As she told me:

> Hawaiians deal in signs, always in signs, yeah. They're not as blunt and forward as people raised in America. They watch for signs. What you do, how you act, what you say, and that's how they judge you. You have to be careful.

Some signs people look for are signs of respect for kūpuna (elders), and your inquisitiveness, or preferably your lack of inquisitiveness. It is a guarantee that many will push you away if you are considered to be too nīele (curious) or maha'oi (forward, pushy).⁹ Typically, a kūpuna will tell you to do something and you do it. Do not or ask why; just do what you are told. The impact that these attitudes can have on research can be a difficult, if not impossible, obstacle to overcome. Two events during my fieldwork revealed the importance of these attitudes.

The first occurred during the preparation for a baby lū'au, which is the celebration of a baby's first birthday and an important event in Hawai'i. Often over 200 people will attend such a party. People rent community centers, hire live bands, and friends, relatives, and caterers provide mass quantities of food and drink. As a prelude to the lū'au, family members and close friends gather almost every night the week before to plan the party, prepare the food, and to just sit, eat, drink, and "talk story"¹⁰ with each other.

During one of these pre-lū'au gatherings at the home of my host family, I made the unfortunate mistake of refusing a beer offered to me by one of the guests. First, there was silence. Then, my refusal was quickly followed by a few jokes about what I would drink and then a quick explanation by the host that while I may look like a Hawaiian I was actually a haole. His explanation was followed by a few comments by the others around the table about how they thought I was Hawaiian, that I looked Hawaiian, and that possibly I was from another island.

As the week progressed, I was asked to run various errands, pick up food, or to help make decorations for the baby lū'au. Although I was asked to help, there were some minor messy chores that I was not asked to do. I really did not notice that I was not asked to do these chores until one evening I insisted on helping prepare the 'opihi. 'Opihi (limpet) is a type of shellfish that is considered a delicacy. Part of the preparation entails removing the meat from the shell with a spoon, which can be messy as the internal contents of the shellfish tended to ooze out of the meat. I was told that I did not need to help because it was such a distasteful and an unpleasant job. Nonetheless, when one of the teenagers did not want to do it anymore, I took her spoon and began to remove the 'opihi from its shell.

When the date of the lū'au arrived I wandered around talking to people, and then sat with friends who had been at the house helping all week. One person at the table was Hinano, the man who had offered me the beer that I had refused. He and his wife were talking to another man when they mentioned that I was from Orange County, California. The man said that he had family living in Fountain Valley, and I said that was really close to where I lived. When I spoke, his mouth dropped open and he just stared at me. I did not know what to think. Had I said something wrong? Had I offended him? Finally Hinano's wife interrupted the horrifying silence and said, "She looks like she's Hawaiian, but when she opens her mouth, we all know," which was followed by laughter. I obviously did not have the appropriate pidgin accent. At this point Hinano said, "But she's all right. I wasn't sure at first, but when she sat down and started shuckin' that 'opihi, then I knew she was okay." This incident was followed by a long conversation on the faults of mainlanders (people who live on the continental United States) and how they do not know how to behave properly. A key problem with mainlanders, in his opinion, was that they were not willing to help at parties, and they never think about bringing enough food or beer to share with everyone. "Mainlanders are stingy," he said, "when they come to a party they only bring enough drink for themselves and when they want more they take from those who brought plenty." Another offering of beer followed his discourse and, of course, I took the beer this time.

The second incident occurred much later in my fieldwork and revealed the interaction between behavior, access to a Native Hawaiian ancestry, and status among islanders. I was invited to a non-profit health organization in a rural area to give a presentation of my work to the staff. This rural area was not part of the original research design (and is not part of the present study). If I was accepted into the community, however, I thought this rural area would make an interesting comparison to the other, more urban island communities where I had already begun working. After my presentation, I was asked to further explain my project and to specify the types of questions I would be asking people. The meeting included me, my Native Hawaiian friend, and three health professionals (two Native Hawaiians, one from the rural area and one from a more urbanized area in the islands, and a white non-Hawaiian woman). After my presentation the health professionals offered their advice on my research. The two Native Hawaiian women suggested that I spend time working in the community, helping in the gardens, volunteering in the clinic, and just hanging around so that the people would get to know me. They also suggested that I avoid being too inquisitive, too nīele. They explained that when a young woman had previously come to the community to conduct a health study, she had gathered a group of the local kūpuna and immediately begun asking questions. The kūpuna, who had things to tell, just sat there with their lips sealed. According to the Native Hawaiian women at the clinic, the other researcher was out of place; not respecting her elders and being inquisitive without first establishing herself by her behavior. In their opinion it would be best for me to spend time helping out in the community before I ever started talking to people about their health. To my surprise, the white woman jumped into the conversation, saying that she did not want me to come in and undermine all their hard work. My friend, who had brought me to the community, had garnered the invitation to the health clinic, and is Native Hawaiian, protested, saying that I would work hard, do anything they wanted; sweep the floor, wash the dishes, whatever. The white woman said while she was sure that I would work hard, there was nothing for me to do. An argument between my friend and the white woman ensued. Because of the tension that was filling the room, the argument seemed to go on for hours, but in reality it lasted for only 15 or 20 minutes. Meanwhile, I sat quietly. While I had no problem helping out in the community and saw it as an extremely valuable experience, I did not want to intrude on the efforts of an already established group. In these moments of disagreement it was clear that someone had crossed the boundaries of proper behavior. What I found most interesting about this whole fiasco was the behavior of the other two women and my friend's reaction to the white woman. The two Native Hawaiian women merely sat there. When the argument was over, the woman from the urban area continued a little bit on the theme of working within the community; the woman from the rural area, however, made no comments either way.

As the incident was recounted to different people, as things of this nature are in small communities, I was able to gain some insight on what had occurred in that unsettling experience. My friend was angry with the "haole" woman for telling her what was going on and how to behave, which is why their argument continued for a prolonged period of time. From my friend's point of view it was inappropriate and offensive for an "outsider," especially a "haole," to tell a Native Hawaiian how to behave. In contrast to the white woman, the rural Native Hawaiian woman was behaving appropriately. I was told that in conflict situations, as a Native Hawaiian, you do not say anything. You wait, then you go home to your elders and tell them what happened, and then follow their advice. The point is to seek advice from your elders and maintain a closed community. The white woman did not act as a Hawaiian should act. She had picked up on the desire by many Native Hawaiians to be left alone, to not have to deal with nīele people who breeze through the community without helping it in any tangible way. Her intentions to protect the community from outsiders may have been admirable, but her actions were very much in line with aggressive haole behavior and even somewhat paternalistic. Native Hawaiians can determine for themselves how open or closed they wish to be, which underscores the argument that developed.

As the weeks went on, we heard conversations and gossip of which the white woman was the focus. She was characterized as a "wanna-be Hawaiian," and as behaving like a "haole." Even though she lived in the community, she was not wholly accepted as a member of the community. Although she was allowed to play gatekeeper through her position at the health center and her contributions to the well-being of the community, she was also criticized for her haole ways.

Both these examples not only show the importance of listening to your elders, of not being too inquisitive, and of behaving as a Hawaiian should, they also show the fluidity and significance of managing one's identity. It was suggested by some that I should let people assume I was Hawaiian, that I belonged, thus avoiding bias and conflict. Part of the problem with that strategy, as I stated at the beginning, is the disjuncture that occurs when people realize you do not fit their a priori category of Hawaiianness. More importantly, it brings up a whole set of ethical concerns. Is letting people assume things about me lying, even though I have no control over what they have assumed? And why should I be afraid to state my own heritage, even though a couple of people made sure that I understood through jokes or direct statements of racial hierarchies that Filipinos are viewed as having lower ethnic status in Hawai'i? Furthermore, what did it mean for me to call myself a Filipino when, besides a biological link to that geographical location, I had no real cultural knowledge, attitudes or behaviors that one would call "Filipino?" And is my father's attachment to Hawai'i, as a person born and raised in Hawai'i, and his subsequent choice to call himself "Hawaiian," which reveals his pride in that aspect of his identity, irrelevant?

This aspect of my identity was less problematic during my fieldwork in southern California. The similarities were that being an active part of the community and helping and sharing were held in high esteem. However, there is an acceptance and even an active effort to include non-Hawaiians in the activities of many of the Hawaiian Civic Clubs. In contrast to my experiences in Hawai'i, less attention was paid to the way I talked or the exhibition of haole behaviors. For example, no one was surprised when I spoke without the appropriate pidgin accent. In addition, although a certain amount of timidity is always considered good behavior, being inquisitive was not looked down upon. Given the range of time that people have lived on the mainland, markers such as language and aggressive or inquisitive behavior do not have the same significance in determining who is Hawaiian and who is not.

In sum, Hawaiian identity is a very self-conscious entity. In making your way through daily life, behaving as a Hawaiian is just as important as having blood ties to pre-contact Hawaiians. There is a rejection of attributes that are associated with haoles or Westerners such as aggressiveness, lack of sharing, and an unwillingness to help with chores no matter how dirty or labor intensive. Ironically, being aggressive in doing the dirty work adds to the likelihood that you will be identified as an insider. It shows that you do not think so highly of yourself that you are unwilling to help, or that you are taking from the community without sharing. Attributes such as listening to your kūpuna, not asking questions, and overall willingness to "go with the flow" are held in high esteem among the people I met. Behaviors are continuously being observed; I was being observed as much as I was observing. Failure to meet the expectations of those who were watching me, expectations based on the way I look, triggered shock, amusement, and social rejection. The visible shifting of categories, however, allowed me to see and understand the boundaries I had crossed. More importantly, the shock, amusement, exclusion, and subsequent inclusion also allowed me to see how the native Hawaiians were managing my identity.

Learning about Hawaiian Health

There are many ways by which specialized Hawaiian knowledge, such as chants, dance, crafts, and medicine, is transmitted throughout the Hawaiian Islands. After many practices had been outlawed after the encounters with foreigners, specialized knowledge was typically transmitted on an apprenticeship basis or kept within families and passed down from one generation to the next. In recent years, with the efforts to revitalize a Hawaiian cultural and national identity and increase the availability and ease by which specialized knowledge is attained, access to knowledge has become more formal. Some of this formal transmission of Hawaiian knowledge takes place in the form of structured classes at community colleges, community centers, and outreach programs, in addition to the highly structured programs offered by universities. While opportunities to acquire Hawaiian knowledge have increased at the local level, for some people these opportunities are also ways to differentiate Hawaiians from non-Hawaiians.

During my field research I attended health classes in Maui and the Big Island. A couple of the classes were offered by nonprofit organizations, others were offered by Hawaiian medicinal practitioners, and for-profit organizations. Two-month-long courses were also provided at the community college in Maui. Some of the classes taught the Wai'anae diet and the importance of eating Hawaiian foods. Another class emphasized the importance of ho'oponopono, conflict resolution, and stress reduction; in other classes we were taught about Hawaiian beliefs of illness causation, cures, and Hawaiian medicinals. All these classes were taught by Native Hawaiians. Furthermore, every kumu (teacher) emphasized the importance of learning from the kūpuna. During their courses they paid respect to the kūpuna who had taught them and encouraged all to listen to the kūpuna so that we would retain as much Hawaiian knowledge as possible.

A very distinct feature of all these courses had not so much to do with the kumu, but rather with the students. The typical class size was about 30 and most of the students ranged in age from 30 to 60 years old. Occasionally students in their early 20s would attend, but that was certainly not the norm. Of those attending these courses only two or three were Hawaiian.[11] The rest of the class was primarily made up of non-Hawaiian whites. With the constant struggle to regain Hawaiian knowledge, revitalize a Hawaiian cultural identity, and the increased opportunities to access Hawaiian knowledge one may wonder why so few Hawaiians chose to attend these courses.

In addition to the time and economic pressures of working multiple jobs, there are a variety of reasons for the low attendance at these formalized learning opportunities. Many of these reasons have to do with local Hawaiians wishing to clearly distinguish themselves from Western ways and the haole population. As Pi'iali'i, who is very active in promoting Hawaiian knowledge and material culture, said in a very straightforward response, "We don't go because the haoles are there." This is a clear rejection of any desire to be in close physical proximity to non-Hawaiians when learning about anything Hawaiian.

Another woman, Nohea, a 49-year-old homemaker, pointed out that given all the other demands of life, such formalized learning is too much work. As she noted:

Well, I think they just want to be themselves, whether Maui, the Big Island, Honolulu, a lot of people are like that, yeah. All different islands but it's the attitude that in the home where you comfortable, go eat, sleep, pay your rent, you happy and that's it. So why study like that?

Her perception is that there is a definite lack of interest in structuring every-day life towards learning in a classroom. Those in the opposing camp, however, are not against learning; rather, they are against the formal setting of a classroom. Formal situations are viewed as spheres of Western control. A Hawaiian attitude to "go with the flow," as one informant stated, lends itself to situations where informal learning is the norm.

Knowledge of Hawaiian tradition and specialized knowledge such as arts and crafts and medicinals primarily took place on an informal basis, that is, learning took place in homes, with kūpuna, close friends and family, and at times when either the kūpuna called or everybody happened to be around. As I was told by some of the kumu, training took place under the direction of the kūpuna and everyone followed, asking no questions, just going with the flow. In other words, the learning of Hawaiian ways still takes place, as it did for early Native Hawaiians, in places that are established as Hawaiian spaces where Hawaiians are in control and practice Hawaiian ways and where the haole typically will not or cannot go. A few people I spoke with suggested that this style of learning was a necessary strategy that allowed them to pass on knowledge that had been outlawed by the missionaries and colonizers.

One example, however, of a situation of formalized learning that has worked well is the Wai'anae Diet Program. In this program classes are held daily for three weeks. A nutritionist from a local Hawaiian health center teaches participants about the health of the pre-contact Hawaiians and their diet. The participants are then taught how to maintain the diet of their ancestors in the contemporary milieu. This diet gives primacy to a Hawaiian way of life. I would argue that creating a Hawaiian space that focuses on Hawaiian ways of knowing and respecting ancestors is a key reason why many people attend this formalized type of learning. This focus has also been a factor in the success of the active outreach programs of other health organizations. As Lehua stated,

> All these health agencies are doing great as far as I find them promoting, well you can see them out promoting to the public. Where before it used to be hush, hush everything. Over here you can go out to the public now and reach 'em. Before everything used to be like you had to be invited into Hawaiian culture to present something. Hawaiians always there to break you out if they don't like what you doing very fast. So really as far as the hui and everything what they do for Hawaiian health is now they advertising it more where the Hawaiians can hear and see and look at results finally and just think about it.

A call to Hawaiians is extended, knowledge is given in a manner that is appropriate, and people are allowed to "just think about it." It is not intrusive or maha'oi. In this case, formal learning is transformed into a Hawaiian space where Hawaiian values and ways are respected and seen as a way of promoting culture and prolonging Hawaiian lives.

Conducting fieldwork in Hawai'i with Native Hawaiians is infused with history that pervades every research encounter. In remembering Hawaiian history we are faced with struggles against hegemonic discourses of capitalism, tourism, and a romanticized "other." These struggles require the exclusionary ideals, behaviors, and spaces that Native Hawaiians claim as their own. In this case, the fieldwork process in the multiple sites not only allowed me to understand how historical and sociopolitical influences shape other cultural identities, it forced me examine how my own cultural identity was in the "process of becoming" throughout the project. As a result of this newfound subjectivity, being disciplined by the expectations of the people I lived with, there is a sense of "fluidarity"—a recognition of the fluidity of our identities and solidarity with those we work with (Nelson 1999). Representations of Island and individual identities are fluid, informed, and impinged on by a history of colonialism, a remembrance of ancestors, and contemporary inequalities and opportunities. And in the midst of this fluidity, we find ourselves in solidarity with the counter-hegemonic movement of Native Hawaiians, with their call to life. Thus, the emphasis on cultural or national identities is more than a representation of alternative ways of being in the world, it is a political statement that clarifies the presence of social and economic inequality and demands that we ask ourselves how we might live.

Endnotes

1. These opinions have long been a part of the historical record, from 1857 and earlier, and a part of other researchers' experiences (see Kame'eleihiwa 1992:20; Friedman 1994, 1997). This question was also raised by a reviewer of one of my research proposals.

2. See the following for more information on the history of displacement and nuclear testing on Bikini atoll. "For the Good of Mankind: A History of the People of Bikini and their Islands" by Jack Niedenthal; PD Jones, From Bikini to Belau; the nuclear colonisation of the Pacific, WRI 1988; RC Kiste, "Identity and relocation; the Bikini case," in M Chapman, ed, Mobility and identity in the Island Pacific, special issue of *Pacific Viewpoint*, 26(1), 1985.

3. Buck's (1993) and Silva's (2004) excellent work shows how throughout the history of Kanaka struggles, hula is used to tell the history stories of Kanaka origins and genealogy. As such, hula is a symbol of resistance to colonial and neocolonial hegemony.

4. Drawing on Anderson (1991 [1983]), Silva argues that Hawaiian newspapers as "print capitalism" forged an "imagined community" of Native Hawaiians.

5. Twenty other interviews were completed with non-Hawaiians (Japanese, Anglo, and Filipino); these interviews will not be discussed in this study.

6. While this household income may seem high in comparison to the U.S. median household income, which is $50,046, in Orange County the median household income is higher at $64,611. The median household income in Hawaii is $56,961 (2000 Census).

7. My father who was born and raised on Maui, had always called himself a Hawaiian. So I always believed that I was part Hawaiian, genealogically speaking. However, years after my father's death and at the beginning of this research, I requested a copy of his birth certificate. On his birth certificate, dated 1927, it stated that both my grandparents were originally born in the Philippines. So my father was raised in Hawai'i, but was not a "Native Hawaiian."

8. Dorinne Kondo (1990) describes similar events during her fieldwork in Japan.

9. Maha'oi, literally meaning sharp temple, to thrust forward one's temples, to be rude or insolent. As my language teacher explained to me, it is like someone with something sharp sticking out of their head and you just want them to get away from you because the sharp thing keeps on hitting and annoying you.

10. *Talk story* is a term used to describe moments when individuals are sitting around and sharing stories with each other. It is a way to both share cultural knowledge and to know people before private, important intentions are revealed.

11. This description applies only to community-level organizations. Personal conversations with university students show that this is not the case at the Manoa and Hilo universities.

3

COMPLICATING HEALTH-SEEKING PRACTICES

Although the impact of foreign influences on Native Hawaiian health was devastating in a historical context, the current health crisis has sparked a renewed sense of urgency. The reportedly poor health of Natives Hawaiians had resulted in a plethora of studies that are set up to understand why this population "fails" to seek medical care when needed and why, when they do seek care, they are so often considered "non-compliant" patients. Many health workers and anthropologists, both within and outside the Native Hawaiian community, are committed to improving the health of Native Hawaiians. However, in structuring questions that rely on implicit Western standards of measurement (such as "failure" or "non-compliance"), these studies are in danger of repeating the all-too-familiar colonial agendas of the past. Whereas Western biomedicine's main goal is to treat illness, its legitimization through ideological, structural, and economic transformations, as evidenced in the Chapter 1, has led to its becoming intertwined with the complex history of the West's domination of Native Hawaiians. Seeking biomedical treatment for poor health then becomes, for many Native Hawaiians, part of the ongoing struggle and negotiation process between the ideologies of the West and re-emerging Hawaiian ideologies.

My purpose in this chapter is to examine the knowledge regarding health-seeking practices, conflicts between biomedical (or "Western medicine," as in the words of my interviewees) and Native Hawaiian medical practices, and how the politics of health-seeking practices reconfigure forms of cultural identity. After briefly describing study participants' health-seeking practices, I explore attitudes towards health, focusing on themes of inclusion and exclusion into the Native Hawaiian community as well as the fluidity with which health is used to represent belonging in the community. Participants' attitudes and actions regarding health and healthcare are seen as part of the on-going political and economic process between dominant models of biomedicine and models of Hawaiian medical knowledge that reflect the fluidity of identity. Although this chapter is primarily focused on the health-seeking practices of on-islanders, both on- and off-islanders view these practices as acts informed by their culture, constrained by structures of biomedical institutions, but nevertheless striving to actively revitalize their own health and their cultural identity within that context.

Debates about Health-Seeking Practices

Health-seeking practices have been and continue to be of interest to public health personnel, physicians, and medical anthropologists. The two most common explanations for why people do not seek medical care or do not follow doctor's orders when they do seek care point to economic and cultural barriers. In the first case, economic obstacles, including lack of money, lack of insurance, and lack of transportation are among the more commonly cited obstacles to care. In the second case, patients' beliefs about health and illness are seen as incongruent with the beliefs of the practitioner. This reported incongruence is further transformed into a problem of lack of knowledge on the part of the patient. If patients were more sophisticated and knew more about medical science, technology, and biology then they would have the same beliefs as the physicians and thus seek care appropriately. This argument has been widely criticized by many scholars because it blames the victim even as it obscures the socioeconomic factors that create barriers to care (Good 1994; Farmer 1999; Baer, Singer, and Susser 2003). These scholars' work demonstrates an integrated approach considering how patient/population beliefs interact with structural factors (Singer and Baer 2007). Thus, in combining the two arguments, one must always take into account both economic obstacles and the beliefs of a population defined as "at risk" (Morgan 1987; Chavez and Torres 1993; Chavez et al. 1995; Chavez et al. 2001). Another argument is that people simply want to feel better and will seek care from any type of practitioner who has the perceived potential to make them feel well (Worsely 1982). It must be noted, however, that typically the standard by which people make choices is measured not by asking why or how people are making the decision to use alternative forms of health care, but rather why are they *failing* to use biomedical care. In the public health literature the issue of failing to seek or follow the directions of biomedical care has been evident in the plethora of articles on non-compliance. Those who fail to seek care from a medical system believed to be more efficacious and hence superior by the dominant society are classified as non-compliant, as pathological, as needing to be fixed (Balshem 1993; Chavez et al. 1995). In order to help non-compliant groups achieve better medical care, the medical gaze is brought to bear on cultural practices that explain "self-destructive" behavior, which in turn pathologizes entire groups and cultural practices, bringing them under greater medical scrutiny (Santiago-Irizarry 2001; Briggs and Mantini-Briggs 2003).

Recognition of Native Hawaiians' low socioeconomic status, their mental and physical health problems, and their "failure" to seek care during the 1960s had resulted in studies that attempted to clarify the problems patients encountered when accessing medical services. Native Hawaiians were defined as a population "at risk," and as a group they were statistically present in every category of "social problem" (Howard 1974). Historically Native Hawaiians were characterized as lazy, unable to adjust, unmotivated, focused on the past (see Fuchs 1961)[1] and thus unwilling to do anything to improve their situation. Contemporary and less negative characterizations have stated that Native Hawaiians do not want to socialize or be an active part of larger society and tend to focus on past history as a "strategy for coping" with the rapidly changing world (Howard 1974; Young 1980). The poor health of Hawaiians has thus been characterized as related to their own behavior, beliefs, and coping strategies, which prevent them from seeking "appropriate" medical care.

The rise of critical medical anthropology and critical studies of the biomedical system, however, has effected a reexamination of the assumptions behind questions pertaining to the source of illness, reasons for seeking care, and the anthropologist's relationship with the biomedical establishment. Scheper-Hughes and Lock (1987) argue that illness episodes can be seen as acts of resistance against subjugation to constrictive social relationships and broader political relationships. Similarly, Ong's 1987 study of Malaysian female factory workers interprets episodes of spirit possession as acts of resistance against the increasing capitalist controls placed on women's lives in the factories. In another example, Martin (1992) argues that in the United States the mechanics of caring for one's body during menstruation, that is, increased bathroom breaks and a slowdown in productivity, can also be viewed as acts of resistance. These studies show the importance of examining the interaction between biological processes and cultural constraints. Biological processes are more than mere illnesses; they can also be tools for critique and resistance in an inegalitarian society.

Viewing illness as partly an act of critique and resistance opens the door for us to think more concretely about issues of non-compliance and "coping strategies" as acts of resistance. Scott's 1985 work on everyday forms of resistance reminds us that resistance is often too narrowly defined. Resistance is not always bold and dramatic; rather, it can take the form of "foot dragging, dissimulation, desertion, false compliance, pilfering, feigned ignorance, slander, arson, sabotage, and so on (xvi)." Using this framework, Balshem (1993) has argued that the working-class community she studied in the United States has made use of these tactics. This group attempted to regain control over their lives and community and against the negative characterizations imposed on them by medical personnel and health educators who brought cancer intervention programs to them. The community resisted recommended lifestyle changes because they felt that their beliefs about cancer and their personal experiences were invalidated by outsiders who alienated them further by labeling accepted behaviors as "bad" lifestyle choices.[2] Similarly Browner and Preloran (2000) argue that Latinas' refusal of amniocentesis after a positive alpha fetoprotein (AFP) screening result can be viewed as an act of resistance and an effort to maintain control of their bodies and their choices. AFP prenatal screening is used as an indicator of potential neural tube defects such as spina bifida and anencephaly. Latinas who refused further testing were characterized as fatalistic because they would not follow physicians' recommendations. A closer examination of Latinas who refused further testing, however, revealed that these women took active steps to change behaviors that they perceived as the cause of the positive AFP. The Latinas' agency stands in stark contrast to any claims of fatalism, especially when compared to other options such a termination of the pregnancy, which is not viewed as fatalistic (Browner and Preloran 2000).

Knowledge of health, from how to become healthy and then maintain health, are infused with constraints and opportunities from Hawai'i's colonial and present political economy of health. Consequently, health and care-seeking are integrated into the processes of cultural identity through acts of resistance and counter-hegemonic moves for sovereignty. Acts of exclusion, references to the past, failures to seek biomedical care, or non-compliance should not be viewed as pathological acts or self-destructive behavior. Native Hawaiians' efforts to obtain health care when ill can been seen in another context, either as acts of resistance or as part of a process of reasserting alternative beliefs about health. In either case, it is imperative to interpret actions through the agency of the individual as opposed to dismissing resistance as passive acts that reveal only lack of knowledge, or writing them off as coping mechanisms or fatalism.[3]

Health-seeking Options in Hawai'i

The many waves of immigrants to Hawai'i over the past 200 years have brought a variety of healing practices, from acupuncture and Filipino herbal remedies to massage techniques and biomedical practices. While many of these practices have remained or merged with other practices, biomedical practices have become the dominant mode of healing on the islands. As discussed in Chapter 1, ideological and structural events, such as the denigration and ultimate outlawing of Hawaiian medicinal practices and the adoption of biomedicine by Hawaiians and Kāhuna to treat illnesses brought by foreigners, contributed to the ultimate predominance of biomedicine. Recent state efforts to make medical care economically accessible have reaffirmed institutional support for biomedicine. This can be seen in the 1974 Hawai'i Prepaid Health Care Act, which attempts to provide near-universal health coverage for all Hawai'i residents.[4] While there are indeed a multitude of alternative forms of health care in Hawai'i, biomedicine receives cultural, economic, and institutional support as the preferred mode of health care. The combined effects of biomedicine as institutionalized through colonization and the neocolonial requirement that biomedicine be used as a condition of insurance structurally situates an ideologically dominant way of thinking about how to be healthy. The ideological and structural focus on biomedicine simultaneously contributes to a devaluing of other styles of medical knowledge and fragments a political conversation that links health, land, and sovereignty in Hawai'i.

If evaluated only in terms of access to insurance and to a regular physician, obtaining biomedical health care is not a problem for most of the people I spoke with in Hawai'i.[5] All the on-islanders I interviewed in Hawai'i had some form of health insurance through their place of employment or through the Hawai'i Medical Service Association (HMSA), the state insurance coverage.[6] In addition, all the on-islanders except one had a regular physician. In California, all but two participants had private insurance paid for by their employers or a combination of employer and individual contributions. Ironically, these two issues, lack of insurance and lack of a regular physician, are most often cited as key reasons why people do not seek medical care (Perez-Stable et al. 1992; Chavez et al. 1995). Although these two issues were not major obstacles to accessing healthcare for the vast majority of people I interviewed, what was apparent was that their health-seeking choices included many other social, cultural, and even economic factors.

Despite the state of Hawai'i's efforts to offer universal insurance coverage, one of the more common reasons on-islanders gave for not seeking health care was money (n=10). Other reasons included being able to take care of the problem themselves (n=3), stupidity (n=2), afraid that the illness was very serious (n=2), laziness (n=1), pride (n=1), and the belief that biomedical medicine does not help anyway (n=1). In total, only 37 percent of the interviewees mentioned any reason for not seeking care. Most participants stated that if they thought they were sick, they would just go to the doctor and that there would be no reason why they would not seek care.

Although money appears at the top of the list of reasons for not seeking health care among those interviewees who provided a reason, the issue of money is not merely about paying bills; rather, it is also about family and responsibility. Money is an issue because of the potential loss of wages resulting from an illness and its impact on the family. Money was also viewed as an obstacle in the context of chronic illness or potential situations in which insurance would not cover all medical bills. Draining family resources in order to pay medical bills was not viewed as the proper way to relate to family. As Ikaika, a man in his late 40s, told me:

> People like to say we're fatalistic because we don't want to go to the doctor when we're dying. But why should we go? The only sure thing in life is death. So if the doctor tells me I got cancer, why should I take all the money my family has worked so hard for? Why should I leave them with a lot of debt and doctor bills to pay? I just want to spend time with my family and make sure everything is right when I leave. So we're not fatalistic, taking care of our family is more important.

The issue of money becomes entwined with concerns about the ramifications of expensive and prolonged care. Although there is universal health coverage, it does not cover all the costs of medical care. To use family resources to benefit the individual places everyone in financial jeopardy, straining already low incomes. Unlike the biomedical point of view, which believes that all medical technology options should be pursued before death takes hold (Koenig 1988; Drummond 2007), Ikaika speaks to the larger issue of death or the acceptance of death as part of the life process. The emphasis on making sure that all is "right" with the family is the overriding concern in health and life. To resist medical treatment that would cause harm, financial or otherwise, is to act according to the life process. For Ikaika, the 'ohana (family), or the care of the family, takes priority.

Attitudes toward Biomedicine

While health insurance coverage and a regular physician make accessing care from biomedical practitioners easier, Native Hawaiian attitudes towards the biomedical system and biomedical practitioners are not always positive. It is relatively common among Americans to criticize the authority of medical practices and knowledge in the United States (Balshem 1993:7); Native Hawaiians are no different in this respect. Their criticism of biomedicine, however, is not reserved to knowledge and practices; in fact, it reveals a certain amount of cynicism about government funding for Native Hawaiian health care, about the quality of the care, and the belief that medical care is ultimately a symbol of difference.

Although increased attention to the poor health statistics and the low socioeconomic status of Native Hawaiians has led to a rise in government funding for research projects, many of the people I spoke with said that they had never seen any direct benefits from these programs. Not surprisingly, a few people were reluctant to speak with me because they were tired of answering questions from outsiders and unsure whether they would see any benefit to their community. People with whom I became close also expressed this sentiment. They told me that they were tired of filling out questionnaires at the doctor's office, tired of talking to researchers who gather knowledge of Hawaiian ways, medicines, and practices, and then use that knowledge to make money selling exploitative books. There was noticeable anger at the perceived profits that outsiders were making from Hawaiian knowledge. As U'ilani, a 40-year-old travel agent, said about all the money and land that is supposed to be used to benefit Hawaiians:

> . . . it depends on how they spend their money. Um, I haven't heard people saying if we lease this land out to a big developer and we charge x amount of dollars then we should start taking that money and building an old folks' home for our kūpuna and . . . then a health care facility. I don't hear that. I hear other things. So it all comes to where their priorities are going to lie. . . . You know they talk about how sick people are but I mean you don't know, they say they need this and they need that. But I haven't seen any plans on it.

There is a clear recognition of the need for a supportive Hawaiian health infrastructure; the sin is in the failure to do anything about those needs with money that is supposed to be used to benefit the community. With nothing concrete that can be held up as a symbol of the benefits of medical or other research in Native Hawaiian communities, research is seen as nothing more than another tool for exploitation.

Even when something concrete is planned for the Hawaiian community, the quality of what is done falls into question. During a conversation with a group of women about the health care available in the community, 'Ikena, a 43-year-old storeowner, clarified the differences between what Native Hawaiians receive and what others receive. She complained about how they, "rich people," donate huge sums of money to get hospitals built in Hawaiian communities, but then the quality of health care is lacking. According to 'Ikena, the quality of health care on the islands does not matter to "rich people," because they do not have to suffer the consequences of poor care. When they are seriously ill, they can afford to fly to the mainland to receive better health care. The only thing "they" are concerned about is their ability to flaunt their "generosity" to the Hawaiian community and their wealth.

However, this is not to say that all health programs are viewed with the same amount of cynicism. Rather, the problem lies with those research and health promotion activities that at the structural level replicate colonial agendas of science and medicine that are aimed at "civilizing" the Natives, ridding them of their own practices in the name of good works. Furthermore, at the relational level these efforts are viewed as neither part of the community nor true exhibitions of caring for the community because researchers neither return their findings nor share who they are as human beings, that is, they do not become an integral part of the community. These efforts are viewed as symbols of difference both in the assumption that the community is unable to provide their own services and in the idea that outsider researchers know better than Natives Hawaiians do about what Native communities need. Furthermore, the services provided by outsiders to be used by the community are not even good enough to be used by the outsiders themselves. Is it any wonder that some are cynical about medical research and services? The final insult is when health providers are left wondering why their services are not being used and it is seen as a non-compliance problem, a problem of the patient, and not of historical and contemporary relationships.

One way that Hawaiians transform the practices of biomedical practitioners and their own cynicism is to insist that practitioners learn how to behave as "proper" Hawaiians. In attending to people's physical needs, a physician grapples with issues of power and legitimacy. Lehua provides an example of Native Hawaiian attitudes towards physicians who would impose their beliefs, and the necessary transformation that must occur before they are accepted as a family's physician:

> Well, at first I thought Dr. Y was crazy because he was one haole. . . . Dr. Y, when he first come down, he come from the mainland. So it was kind of hard for him to adjust to the rest of us. Oh, he did, and now he's so down to earth you wouldn't believe it. Yeah, so, but he's cool, and he opens his mind to a lot of traditional Hawaiian medicines, the old Hawaiian ways of doing that. It took him years to learn but finally he knows. . . . He usually let us talk story first, because that's the way it is with the Hawaiian people. You gotta talk story first. And he says "whatever you guys decide," he'll go with it. You know, he's been here too long to know, you no push a Hawaiian. You let them come to you. You cannot just go to them.

The physician's acceptance not only of Hawaiian medicines, but also of a Hawaiian way of practicing medicine, which includes an approach to doctor-patient relations that entails providing a space for patients to "talk story," are key to his acceptance by this Hawaiian family. Lehua's insistence that the physician behave properly and ultimately effect a change in his attitudes can be viewed as resistance, a reassertion of Hawaiian values into biomedicine, and an effort to negotiate competing models of practicing health care.

Hawaiian Practices/Practitioners

Biomedicine is not the only source of care available in the Islands. Most of the people I interviewed reported having a positive view of Hawaiian medicines. Most continue to seek care from Hawaiian practitioners and have maintained knowledge of medicinal practices in their families. Of those participants who completed structured interviews, 75 percent noted that Hawaiian medicinal practices were good and had something to offer in terms of curing illness and maintaining health.

While several people on-island mentioned having difficulty finding Hawaiian practitioners, 68 percent of the people I interviewed had sought care from a Hawaiian practitioner. All those who sought care from Hawaiian practitioners used either a lā'au lapa'au (herbalist) or a lomi-lomi (massage) practitioner, or both.[7] The types of ailments they sought care for ranged from trouble with spirits, 'opu huli (turned stomach), psoriasis, broken or dislocated bones or joints, and back problems. People noted their preference for Hawaiian practitioners when seeking relief of stress and to relax their muscles, which explains the high use of lomi-lomi. The only other alternative type of health practitioner that interviewees were likely to consult was chiropractors. None of the interviewees had visited other types of alternative health practitioners, such as acupuncture or acupressure providers. Also, no one mentioned using naturopaths or massage therapists other than lomi-lomi.

In California, off-islanders were less likely to have sought care from a Hawaiian practitioner because of the lack of Hawaiian medicinal practitioners in the region. Most of the off-islanders told me about local Native Hawaiians who were biomedical physicians, but they were hard-pressed to name even one Hawaiian medical practitioner practicing in California. If they used Hawaiian medicine, it was because they had visited the island, and a friend or relative had taken them to see the kahuna for their ailments. Like the on-islanders, none of the off-islanders had visited other types of alternative practitioners on the mainland.

Home remedies were another source of health care utilized by some families. Some of the Hawaiians I spoke with mentioned that they had learned and passed on knowledge of Hawaiian medicines and massage techniques through their family. Ten of the on-islanders (29 percent) stated that either they or someone in their family has knowledge of Hawaiian medicines and practices. When feeling ill, they often felt competent enough to treat the illness themselves with

Hawaiian practices or they went to see a family member who had knowledge of local medicinal practices.

One other option that the interviewees have when choosing health care is to rely on family networks. All except three of those interviewed had relied on family networks to provide support when they were ill. These networks were made up of immediate family members and did not draw on extended family such as cousins, aunts, or uncles. Relying on family members is one option that allows people to stay out of the biomedical system. Native Hawaiians are not less likely to seek health care; rather, they choose to rely on individuals who are viewed as part of the community. Ka'ala, for example, a 39-year-old social worker, states the connections between diet, health, economics, and family ties that underlie Hawaiian help-seeking patterns:

> I think of it in terms of generations. There were a lot of changes in the Hawaiian society and the diet changed. Then when the diet changed, that's when a lot of the people's physical health started to be affected. And I think Hawaiians maybe don't seek out medical help from doctors as much as other people do. They tend to rely on alternative care, things within the family. You know try to see if there are other people in the family that can help them. Uhm . . . —*instead of going to the doctor?*— Yeah yeah.—*So it's not that they don't seek care at all*—No. And I wouldn't say it's because they don't care about themselves because I think they do. I think economics too has a lot to do with it. Like even the food, you know, because of the things that are less expensive to buy. The Hawaiians generally have big families and little money, so they buy the canned stuff that . . . maybe is easier, is cheaper and easier to stretch and feed a lot of people.

In Ka'ala's opinion, Hawaiian health-seeking practices are not a simple matter. She contextualizes the problem by citing a change in the diet of Hawaiians as being the ultimate source of illness. The solution entails a heavy obligation and reliance on family to care for one another and to share whatever food is attainable. Diet, for many Hawaiians, is not just about eating right. Chapter 5 examines the role of diet in greater detail, but suffice it to say that diet and the change in diet among Hawaiians is about depopulation, the loss of Hawaiian social structure, and the loss of land. Health problems that Hawaiians suffer are seen as a consequence of the presence of outsiders who effected a change in the food that is available to Hawaiians. Caring for the family extends to the type of food that Hawaiians choose to consume, that is, foods that are relatively inexpensive and that can be stretched, even if that food may be less nutritious than traditional foods. Seeking health care, in part, is about creating definitions about who belongs in the community, or who demonstrates their Hawaiian identity through caring and sharing.

In addition to the practices that are used as symbols of Hawaiian identity (insider versus outsider), there are obstacles to accessing care from Hawaiian practitioners. When I refer to Hawaiian medical practitioners I am specifically speaking about lāʻau lapaʻau (herbalists) and providers of lomi-lomi (massage), the two forms of care commonly used by interviewees. These types of practices are not exclusive. A practitioner may be skilled as both lāʻau lapaʻau and lomi-lomi but may emphasize one practice more than the other. These are also not the only types of Hawaiian medical practices,[8] but they are the ones most commonly used, along with to hoʻoponopono (conflict resolution). People typically use Hawaiian medical practices because they have knowledge that was passed down through the family, or they view Hawaiian practices as inherently better, or because Western medicine has not met their needs. Reasons for not using Hawaiian practitioners most often have to do with trouble accessing the practitioners, primarily the fact that insurance does not cover care by Hawaiian practitioners, or that people do not know where to find a reputable practitioner.

One reason that people gave for not seeking care from Hawaiian practitioners is that they do not know how to locate a Hawaiian practitioner or one that they feel they can trust. When asked if she would ever seek out care from a Hawaiian practitioner, Mokihana, a 28-year-old college student who also works three jobs to support herself and pay for her education, stated:

> I guess so, but they're not readily available. To me it feels like, you know, like the other doctor's right there. I can just go make an appointment for this. For this I don't know, I don't know who to contact. I don't know where to go. When it's more hard for me to get there, 'cause I'm so busy, I usually won't go. I just go there [to the biomedical doctor] 'cause I can usually get my appointment. Get in and get my stuff and I'm done.

It is not only a matter of not knowing where to go, seeking care is also tied up with the ease of using biomedical care. For the same reasons that finding a regular biomedical physician is an obstacle to health-seeking (not knowing where to go, not knowing who to trust, the time it takes to see the physician) the difficulty of finding a Hawaiian practitioner is also an obstacle to seeking care from that type of practitioner.

I would not argue, however, that choosing not to seek care from a Hawaiian practitioner is done without self-reflection. As Kūpaʻa, a 41-year-old single father with four children, stated:

> Right now it seems so convenient for me to see a regular doctor you know. But then I think there's more respect [with Hawaiian practices] and I need to educate myself and find out what's there.

The hegemony of biomedicine leads to a partial erasure of knowledge about where to seek Hawaiian medical care. This erasure takes place, in part, through the combined effects of the institutionalization of medicine through forms of practitioner licensing as suggested in Chapter 1, and the determination of what practices medical insurance will pay for. This partial erasure leads to an estimation of what medicine is "convenient" in the contemporary milieu and an ideological skepticism of the efficacy of non-biomedical practices and consequently a limited number of and knowledge about where to find practitioners of Hawaiian medicine. What it also suggested by Kūpaʻa is that overcoming or resisting the convenience of biomedical care is a matter of respecting Hawaiian practices and, by educating himself, gaining self-respect. This desire by many younger Hawaiians to seek the medical knowledge of the ancestors suggests that they are embracing the revitalization movement as a viable option for their lives. In other words, using Hawaiian medicine entails a way of thinking about the world and the body; it is more than just a convenience. As Hauʻoli, a very outgoing 60-year-old woman, stated:

> I've talked to a lot of older folks and had some really good stories from them about people who have been treated. . . . I don't think you can just say "Oh, Hawaiian medicine is going to work," and just do it. I think you really have to do it in the traditional Hawaiian way. And that's a very spiritual kind of experience. It's not just getting medicine and taking it.

Thus, according to Hauʻoli, Hawaiian medicine should be used only when you have the right attitude, a Hawaiian attitude, which includes an appropriate set of cultural assumptions and understandings. The spiritual issue that Hauʻoli is referring to in this quote is lōkahi; the integration of body, spirit, emotion, and healing powers or mana that comes from the land. Healing, again, is more than attending to the symptoms. These quotes show the emerging revitalization of Hawaiian practices and the impact they have in reconfiguring health-seeking choices. For the most part, people want to feel better (physically and culturally), but there are other issues such as convenience (in the context of culturally imposed social and economic demands), dueling subjectivities (between the hegemonic support of biomedicine and the counter-hegemonic insertion of Hawaiian values and medicine), and the economics that play a part in their decisions.

Another obstacle to seeking care from Hawaiian practitioners comes from the insurance institutions. Some interviewees (39 percent) used a combination of biomedical practitioners and Hawaiian practitioners when dealing with illnesses. Their primary motivation for using both, however, generally had to do with the requirements of insurance companies and efficacy of the practitioner, not the severity of the illness. Circumstances that led to the use of both kinds of practitioners included whether or not the illness required biomedical technology, and thus a reluctant use of insurance and all the bureaucratic red tape that it entails, or whether or not the illness could be treated by Hawaiian practitioners. Mililani, a 38-year-old woman, discussed her experience with back problems that prevented her from walking and kept her out of work for months. Her case is an example of how many Native Hawaiians end up consulting both biomedical and Hawaiian practitioners:

> Well it's an insurance thing. I have to go to the doctors first. I went to the doctors just for insurance purposes, the job. And it wasn't working but they still wanted me for go on therapy and take all these drugs they were giving me. Well, I did it on my own. I just went on my own and I went to see Kahuna M [a Hawaiian practitioner]. But I still have to do what the insurance wanted me to do. And six months out of work, no can, no can. So I went to see Kahuna M so he could fix me up. And he did. And then I went back to work afterwards and I still working. You know, walking anyway.

While the issue of efficacy is central to Mililani's justification for using a Hawaiian medical practitioner, it is not the main issue that she focuses on in telling me about her injury. Instead, she situates her agency within the constraints of the insurance company. Drugs and physical therapy are interventions that the insurance company wanted, not something that she wanted for herself. The implication of her experience is that the insurance companies, the outsiders, do not know what will restore her health. She, on the other hand, knows who can restore her health. In detailing the strict management of her body by the insurance company and the ultimate effectiveness of the treatment she received from Kahuna M, Mililani resists the hegemony of biomedicine and offers us knowledge that reveals another path to health. This view was expressed again when talking with a retired couple, Kane and Wahine U'i, in their home. Their conversation reveals the management of the body through insurance companies, and their resistance to that discipline:

> (Kane) If it's an insurance injury then I gotta go to the insurance doctor, that's the white man doctor. Where there's nothing to be public, for instance, you don't have to bring the sick paper, then you go to the Hawaiian doctor.

> (Wahine U'i) Usually the Hawaiian doctor suggests that you go to the white man doctor first for any x-rays or anything like that.

> (Kane) But don't put the cast on it.

> (Wahine U'i) Yeah, but don't put white man medicine. And then you go back you tell them what the doctor told you. And then they take it from there.

(Kane) See I broke my knee and went to Dr. YY, everyday, everyday.

(Wahine Uʻi) Because we were going to the doctor and they couldn't bring the bruise or the swelling down. His leg just getting bigger and bigger. So she [Hawaiian practitioner] put Hawaiian medicine, yeah. She just wrapped up and three days the swelling went away.

I heard about many similar encounters from other people I talked with. Their preference is to use Hawaiian medicine, but they are prevented by the requirements of the insurance companies. These individuals end up spending their time traveling back and forth to different practitioners, first determining whether or not the illness will be covered by insurance, filling out paper work, and finally going to the Hawaiian practitioner. Experiences such as these reinforce the belief that Hawaiian medicine can be more efficacious in many instances, but most insurance companies do not support its use.[9] For those who know how to access Hawaiian practitioners, the irritating process of filling out insurance papers and perpetual visits to the doctor's office are examples of biomedicine or "white man's medicine." Biomedical experiences stand in stark contrast to the care they received from practitioners of Hawaiian medicine, who, in their experience, treat illness quickly and effectively. As one lomi-lomi practitioner said to me "they [biomedical practitioners] don't want to take care of things, they just want you to keep on coming back." The insurance companies and the biomedical physicians are seen as "public," as outside the private community of Native Hawaiians. Insurance companies are something that must be dealt with but there is very little faith that they will pay for care that is needed, care that is appropriate for Native Hawaiians. In drawing out the management of their bodies and health by insurance companies, they feature the regulatory and disciplinary facets of Foucault's biopolitics. Yet, in their pluralistic use of both forms of medicine, they move through and beyond resistance to the discipline of biomedicine and its institutions and into a revitalization of Hawaiian knowledge that is essential for maintaining health in the contemporary milieu.

The Purity of the Hawaiian Way

The revitalization of health and medical practices, however, is contrasted with the historical hegemony of biomedicine through depopulation and denigration that led to the loss of people and knowledge (Chapter 1). In returning to the history of what was lost, Native Hawaiians can craft a framework for the necessity of alternative knowledges. Thus, a Hawaiian knowledge of medicine and health must not only be efficacious, it must also reveal and contest the integrated workings of biomedicine and capitalism. Mililani's discussion of her grandparents' health compared to her own health moves us through loss, a critique of capitalism, and then an imperative for returning to a Hawaiian way of living:

> We have bad health more now than our grandparents had before. 'Cause it's like they had to take care of themselves with herbs. Which today we don't have the herbs because they poison the herbs. So they gotta live off drugs. And think, you gotta pay for those things. What you grow from your 'āina (land) you don't have to pay for. But now you gotta live off drugs to live and I think that's, that's sick. It's a harder life now to me. 'Cause everything costs yeah, now, and then never for them. But they don't believe in the Hawaiian ways of healing. The Western, the Western, they don't believe in the Hawaiian ways of uhm . . . you know when you get sick you go to the ocean and you heal yourself in the ocean, or eat certain kinds of leaves from the land, they don't believe in those. And the Hawaiians live more long then, than they do now.

The dual critique that Mililani illustrates is in the contrast between efficacy and belief of biomedical and Hawaiian medicines, which is underpinned by the progress of capitalism. The Western medical community's failure to believe in Native Hawaiian medicines and its ultimate belief in its superiority to Hawaiian ways is manifested in permitting medicinal herbs to be destroyed, and blocking access to using the land or ocean for health or many other practices. Moreover, both insurance, which is linked to employment, and the use of prescription drugs, require money. Modern drugs replace Hawaiian herbals, which increases the economic ties of Native Hawaiians to a Western or capitalist lifestyle. In sum, medical practices are viewed as issues of control: control over who defines what is good for restoring and maintaining health and their use of technologies, that in this case pollute Hawaiian medicinals, to regulate and support the hegemony of biomedicine.

As argued by Singer (1981), the counter-hegemonic thinking similar to Mililani's contention that a Native Hawaiian lifestyle is viewed as purer than the life that the West and biomedicine offers is shared by dominated groups in the context of industrial capitalism, such as the Black Hebrews in Israel described in his study. Discourses of better physical and psychological ways of living through specific cultural knowledges give rise to the development of stronger communities by excluding the dominant capitalist system. For Native Hawaiians, the 'āina, the plants obtained from the land are deemed pure, they provide a more "natural" way of restoring health. Like Mililani, Lani, a 49-year-old volunteer receptionist, agrees that the medicines of the West are only making things worse:

> I wish we could go back to the Hawaiian way of doing things. Sometimes it's a lot more, to me it's a whole lot better. . . . Sometimes the medicine [biomedical

medicine] makes it worse instead of better. You know and their, the Hawaiian way of doing things is the pure way of doing stuff. You know, both sides have good and bad but I think our Hawaiian ways are a whole lot better. So we still have to fight to preserve our society.

We are provided with an alternative vision that locates the path to health in a Hawaiian heritage. This path becomes salient through their experience of Hawaiian medical practices, and their ultimate decision to use one type of healing over another depending on the type of disease. Decisions are framed as issues of outsiders (Western medicine or white man's medicine) versus insiders (Hawaiian medicine). Although biomedical healing may be more convenient and may or may not work, Hawaiian healing is significant in its ability to create cultural and psychological, and ultimately political, links to a state of health.

Health-seeking Practices, Biomedical Hegemony, and Fluid Identities

Understanding health-seeking practices under conditions of medical pluralism is not simply a matter of choosing between economics and culture. As we have seen, many people are concerned about both issues and often seek biomedical care because it is perceived as "easier" and ubiquitous. However, Native practitioners may be more difficult to find, and/or individuals feel they do not have sufficient knowledge to engage in Hawaiian practices. On the flip side, Hawaiians do not seek biomedical care or follow doctors' instructions for a variety of reasons. The state's universal health coverage plan appears to partially negate the argument that money concerns prevent Hawaiians from seeking care. Despite universal health coverage, Hawaiians still have the poorest health statistics in the state. So why then do Hawaiians choose not to seek care from biomedical practitioners? Why do they choose family as their source of care? Why do some still use lāʻau lapaʻau and lomi-lomi? As we have seen, part of the answer still has to do with economics and the hassle of dealing with the insurance companies. Biomedicine and its institutions represent the "other" for the people I spoke with. Discourses of biomedicine and its historical links to the devaluing of Hawaiian medicine, combined with its intimacy with capitalism represent spaces that are not amenable to Hawaiians or their ways of knowing. Their critique of capitalist intrusions is bolstered by the belief that the medicine provided by the West is not as good as the medicine Native Hawaiians could provide for themselves. These views extend into the practices that reveal caring for and maintaining ties with the ʻohana, as well as the demands on and efforts by biomedical physicians to incorporate these values into their practice. Those people and practices that do not exhibit these values reify the desire to maintain community boundaries. The question posed here, however, is whether Native Hawaiian health care choices are merely a way of "coping" with the influences of the West and biomedical intrusions? Or is a focus on the past a form of resistance, a means to revitalize an identity that challenges a Western model of health? Is there a new a model, a new guide for action towards what Hawaiian health can be? Examining health practices as a search for well-being and a struggle over ideologies as a way to reconfigure identity, rather than as "failings" or "non-compliance" provides a richer description of the complexities of cultural attitudes towards health care. Health practices are effective representations of identity because they reveal the conflicts between capitalism and Hawaiian sovereignty over defining the proper way to live. Moreover, these examinations reveal how Native Hawaiians engagement in all forms of medical care creates contexts where we can see how they challenge representations of their identity as well as craft stronger representations of their own position. These shifts between contesting biomedicine, transforming the practices of biomedicine, and promoting Hawaiian medicine provide insights into the fluidity of cultural identity as integral to transforming political processes. Health as a symbol of cultural identity is sometimes used to represent the values of caring for the family; at other times it shows strength in resisting institutional constraints on individual behaviors. More often than not, however, in the contemporary moment it is used to show the revival of the relationship of Native Hawaiians to their ancestors. Viewing previous Hawaiian practices as pure or as more "natural" provides Native Hawaiians with motivation for action. "We must still fight to preserve our society" is a call not only to challenge Western assumptions of health and medicine, it is also a way to remember the ancestors. It is a call for a "pure" lifestyle that is modeled after a prescription of life for earlier generations of Native Hawaiians.

Endnotes

1. See King (1987) and Merry (1998 n.p.) for good historical description and analysis of negative characterizations of Hawaiians.
2. Balshem recommends that we should still promote healthy behaviors such as low-fat diets and exercise, but that these recommendations should be made in a non-judgmental manner.
3. Some researchers also argue that subjugated populations may internalize the dominant society's expectations. Hence, they fulfill the stereotype and do not meet the standardized criteria of the dominant society. For example, Steele (1995) has shown that African Americans score better on intellectual tests when told that the researchers were merely asking for their opinion. In contrast, the same group scored

poorly when told they were taking a test. Steele refers to this phenomenon as "test anxiety." In sum, it is the stereotypes of African Americans' ability to do well on intellectual tests that have been internalized and that create so much anxiety that the individuals do poorly on tests.

4. As of 2003, 10 percent of the population in Hawai'i was uninsured (United States Census 2003) compared to 21 percent in California and 16 percent nationwide (Brown et al 2005). The 21 percent of uninsured in California include those who were uninsured for part of 2003 year and throughout the whole year.

5. The intent of the Health Care Act was to provide health insurance to everyone. There are many who fall through the gaps, such as self-employed individuals (Burke 1992).

6. The only other large insurance provider on the islands is Kaiser Permanente; only one interviewee had insurance coverage through Kaiser.

7. Five people sought care from a lā'au lapa'au practitioner. Seven people sought care from a lomi-lomi practitioner. Five people sought care from both la'au lapa'au and lomi-lomi practitioners. Eight people sought care from one person who practiced both lā'au lapa'au and lomi-lomi.

8. Some other Hawaiian medicinal practices include Kāhea—healing by calling out to the spirits. HāHā—the practice of being able to diagnose by touching. Ha'i Ha'i iwī—a specialist in setting bones. Pā 'ao'ao—a specialist in very small children.

9. Some agencies under the Hawaiian Health Care System or Papa Ola Lokahi will assist individuals in obtaining insurance and providing referrals to Native Hawaiian health practitioners. These physicians may or may not integrate Hawaiian medical practices into their treatment.

4

VARIATIONS IN DEFINITIONS OF HEALTH

Native Hawaiian and biomedical healing practices are two facets of a complex set of social relationships that give insight into power struggles, transformations in the valuing of specific types of knowledge, and cultural representations of health. As discussed in Chapter 3, focusing on the meanings and experiences associated with individuals who seek care from Native Hawaiian or biomedical practitioners illuminates the relationships between the ideological dominance of biomedicine and structural support through insurance institutions and the creation of obstacles for accessing Hawaiian medicine. In this chapter I examine on- and off-islanders' definitions of health. For the people I spoke with, the variations in health-seeking practices and definitions of health are partly influenced by an individual's social position. For example, the paucity of people practicing Native Hawaiian medicine off-island understandably translates into less use as well as less knowledge about those practices. The issue of access to health care is both an economic and an availability problem that is manifested in differences in knowledge about the meaning of health. As on- and off-islander Kanaka Maoli are influenced by the hegemony of biomedicine on the one hand and the counter-hegemony of a revitalized Hawaiian view of health on the other, their knowledge and practices move along a spectrum that includes physical and social perspectives on health.

Native Hawaiian definitions of health are a mix of perspectives: some biomedical and some that incorporate many of the historical events discussed in Chapter 1. For many of the people I spoke with, this revitalized definition is the embodiment of contemporary and historical struggles over land and knowledge. The inclusion of historical struggles in this definition facilitates a sense of shared community and a position from which to be a "Hawaiian," to experience individual and group identity. Moreover, as Native Hawaiian definitions of health become the embodiment of struggle, the alternate meanings contest and complicate taken-for-granted explanations of experiences and expectations for what the future might hold. In the dispute over the dominant model of health, which is aimed at ridding the body of disease and so focuses primarily on individual practices while ignoring the social and historical context,—we are provided with the foundation for a culturally meaningful alternative of health and identity for Hawaiians. An examination of alternative definitions can foreground the complexities encountered in resisting hegemonic ideologies. Health, like the body and even like the land, is often taken by larger society to be natural, that is, its composition, functioning, and existence are presumed to be the essential and untainted components of life (Foucault 1979; Scheper-Hughes and Lock 1987; Turner 1996). It is through this constructed naturalness that the relationship between health, body, land, and the exercise of power is obscured, making way for the dominance of biomedicine and capitalist production (Foucault 1973; also see Introduction and Chapter 1). Through an examination of alternative definitions of health that emphasize the exercise of power in constructing the meaning of land, health, and body, the pre-eminence of Enlightenment and biomedical views is decreased and attention can be directed towards the effects of social conditions on health. Simultaneously highlighting the historical and social conditions for health reveals the importance of context for cultural identity and underpins the critiques of health inequalities.

This chapter examines how specific constructs and contexts give meaning to the general concept of health. In addition, I elaborate on how some elements gain greater importance in revitalization of Native Hawaiian identity and as a critique of capitalism and inequality. In thinking about the definition of health for a CMA approach, Singer and Baer (2007) extend Kelman's 1975 distinction between experiential and functional health. Kelman noted that experiential health was an individual's ability to function and have a sense of tranquility; functional health, however, was an individual's ability to complete tasks necessary for a capitalist mode of production. Although the functional definition of health acknowledges capitalism's need for a particular kind of body for its work, Singer and Baer argue that this definition did not include the broader structural barriers that can impinge on both functional and experiential health. As such, Singer and Baer's definition includes "the basic material and nonmaterial resources that sustain and promote life at a high level of satisfaction" (2007:64). This definition incorporates an acknowledgment of the social production of health and definitions of health as they are manifested in particular socio-historical contexts.

As we begin to elaborate on Native Hawaiians' knowledge and definitions of health, the historical and contemporary contextual facets of power relationships that affect basic material and non-material resources are revealed. These power relationships are manifested in knowledge struggles as definitions of health are at times similar to the hegemonic ideologies (a functional view of health), but they are also counter-hegemonic in that they appropriate and then critique functional, Enlightenment, and biomedical views. At the most general level, the functional level, on- and off-islanders defined health in similar ways. However, when thinking about what it meant to be a healthy Hawaiian, some people thought back to the livelihood of the pre-contact Hawaiians, while others thought of their contemporary relatives. The differences in how far people thought back in the timeline was often associated with the degree to which health was framed as a social or individual responsibility. A social responsibility framing linked historical and contemporary inequities (depopulation, unequal access to land and food) and held up the ancestors as an integrated model for how to live life. In contrast, the view of health as an individual responsibility did not forefront social and economic inequities as part of a production of health. This view held that engaging in practices that are presumed to be available to all allows one to live as a Native Hawaiian. Both views, however, reflected an interest in remembering, preserving, and practicing Hawaiian culture. When health was defined as an individual responsibility, memories of ancestors' practices such as hula, language, music, family gatherings and festivals were important for identity but were not part of what constituted health. Health as a social responsibility, however, was defined through its link to memories of the practices just mentioned as well as the ancestors' ties with the land, and knowledge that supported the view of the purity of pre-contact lifestyles. Connections that people made to the land and ancestors, or social and individual responsibility for health was often linked to their status as transnationals who were trying to make connections to a place away from the 'āina (land).

Many have recognized the role of technology (i.e., telephones, rapid air travel, the Internet) for transnational communities in maintaining links and weaving the symbols of their "homeland" with their experiences in their new place of residence (Rouse 1985; Morton Lee 2003). These communities, however, must also negotiate the lifestyle and discourse of the dominant culture in which they live (Basch et al. 1994). As Hall (1994) noted, we must attend to the place in which the reconstruction of a cultural identity occurs because it influences the meanings and symbols chosen to represent that cultural identity. This contextualization of representation creates a space to think about how cultural identities are, as Hall argues, a matter of "being" as well as a matter of "becoming." Identity belongs to the future as much as to the past (p. 394). Thinking of identity as a state of becoming allows us to see both the importance of a shared common origin, the transformations that create differences between those who have remained in the "homeland" and those who have left by choice or by force, and the larger structural forces that impinge on or facilitate access to resources that inform individual subjectivities. Thus, following a pattern similar to that of health-seeking practices, definitions of health reflect a positioning of identity relative to biomedical practices and Native Hawaiian medical practices.

The analysis for this chapter and Chapter 5 reveals the importance of context in the struggle over the meaning of models of health and shows that some cultural symbols are not as portable (land) as other cultural symbols (hula). Land as a cultural symbol can have specific meanings attached to it, such as the "homeland," the place of the ancestors, or as the embodiment of the gods (e.g., Pele). These are ideals and values that may travel with transmigrants. Yet, in the postcolonial era land is difficult to access because of "ownership" struggles and distance, so the land-health connection does not take on the same relative importance when the separation is great. When living away from the 'āina one cannot literally bathe in the waters or cultivate the land of the ancestors because the land is not portable, thus these practices result in different meanings for off-islanders. The different meanings of these portable and immovable symbols give rise to different ways of integrating views on how to be healthy and honor one's ancestors. The meaning of health, for on- and off-islanders, reflects a fluidity wherein identity and a potential counter-hegemonic view of health are positioned relative to Hawaiian ancestors, colonial domination, popular health information, and peers who live on opposite shores.

General Views on Health

What it means to be healthy for on- and off-islanders encompasses many popular and scientific beliefs about the body and illness. Similar to Crawford's 1984 findings on middle-class American constructions of health, when asked to describe a healthy person, many people I spoke with responded with answers that may constitute the attributes of a functional and, at times, an experiential view of health such as the "ability to work," "to be energetic," "to exercise," "eating a healthy diet," and "having a positive attitude". It is important to emphasize that most respondents focused on a functional view of health, what it means to *be* healthy, and very rarely on an abstract definition of health. For example, Ipo, who has lived on Maui his whole life and leads a somewhat active life, had this to say:

> I think you gotta have exercise in your life to be healthy. Uhm, eating the right
> foods, cutting back on red meat. I wish I was vegetarian to tell you the truth, but

I got a hard time to get away from meat. A healthy person has to eat fruits and vegetables and I think exercise is the main thing.

This is a common refrain that you hear in the United States today; eating a balanced diet, avoiding too much red meat, and exercising regularly are the basics in order to be healthy. These are things that a person must do in order to be healthy and to function properly in today's society. Likewise, Kupuna Nani, who is 63 and works on the assembly line in a small factory in California, viewed being healthy as the ability to move around, as she said:

Healthy. For one thing to be healthy means not feeling bad or hurting or uhm, able to walk. . . . So health is you know, exercising and uhm even if it's stupid, you're old you can't do barbells, but even just walking. Walking helps. I noticed that yesterday, coming back, my husband can hardly wait to go home and put his feet up. I'm all, "I could go another mile." I didn't tell him that. But that's what health is, when you get older it's just not hurting because a lot of people wake up with aches and pains.—*So exercise and being active is* . . . —yeah because it's like an old, a nut and bolt. If you let it go it gets rusty. But if you shake it ever so often and oil it, it'll be there for years.

To talk about health is to talk about independence, a shared goal in the contemporary United States. Similar to Ipo's views, every example of being healthy that Kupuna Nani gave was related to her either being able to continue doing her work (things that the other older women could not do) or outlasting her husband in terms of physical endurance. It is a functional view of health, a state of being able to do certain things and not just a state of being or experience. She furthers her image of health by drawing on the metaphor of the body being a machine, implicitly pointing to the understanding that health is under the control of the individual, and that by caring for and providing the proper maintenance measures you can maintain the body for years.

These attributes of a healthy person are common knowledge within the United States, particularly the importance of eating right: decreasing your consumption of red meat and increasing your consumption of fruits and vegetables, and most importantly the ubiquitous, yet poorly defined, need to exercise (Crawford 1984; Whorton 1988; Leichter 1997; Lupton 1997). Table 4.1 lists the attributes of a healthy person as derived from the semi-structured interviews. One could argue that these are the responses you would receive from most people living in the United States, and that they are representative of the ideal of individualism and the belief that health is a personal responsibility.

Further analysis of these descriptions reveals two contrasting definitions of health. The first is based on statements of exclusion, opposition to values from the

Table 4.1.   Attributes of a Healthy Person Hawaii and California Comparison

Item Mentioned	% HI (n = 35)	Item Mentioned	% CA (n = 17)
Eating right	77	Eating right	80
Exercise	60	Exercise	73
Being able to be active, energetic	46	Being able to be active, energetic	47
Having a positive attitude	34	Little stress in life	23
Little stress in life	26	Having a balance between emotional, spiritual, and physical life	12
Having a balance between emotional, spiritual, and physical life	20	Having a spiritual life	12
Having a spiritual life	17	Getting enough rest	12
Salt water cleanse	9	Getting an annual check-up	12
Getting enough rest	9	Positive about self and heritage	12
Eating food from the land	9	Taking care of personal appearance and hygiene	12
Not having to worry about illness	6	Not smoking	12
Good family relationships	3	Being in beautiful surroundings	6
Having confidence	3	Good family relationships	6

Note: Percentages do not add up to 100 because each respondent may mention more than one item each.

West, the purity of Hawaiian ways, and attachments to pre-contact Hawaiians' views and practices, as currently conceived through revitalization efforts. This interpretation promotes a particular view of health and cultural identity that is critical of colonial intrusions—from the ideological devaluation of Hawaiian knowledge, to the introduction of deadly diseases and the taking of Hawaiian lands. The second meaning draws on images of individual control of the body. These contrasting views of health, control of the body versus control of the land, take center stage as points of debate in the meaning and achievement of health.

Off-islanders cited similar general elements for being healthy as those cited by on-islanders. Both groups mentioned eating the right foods (77 percent on-islander versus 80 percent off-islander) and exercise (60 percent on-islander versus 73 percent off-islander), as keys to being healthy (see Table 4.1). The appearance of these items at the top of the on-islander list demonstrates the prevalence of these functional lifestyle beliefs that emanate from both the public health literature and popular U.S. culture (Lupton 1997). Yet, as I will argue through the remainder of this chapter, off-islanders associate a different set of meanings to these two general concepts than do on-islanders. For off-islanders, eating right and exercising have more to do with the importance of appearance and the main-tenance of the physical body, and with the ability to be independent than with the maintenance of a relationship with the land. As such, this view does not acknow-ledge the historical and contemporary power relationships that create conditions for good or poor health. It does, however, correspond to Kelman's 1975 functional view of health. However, in off-islanders' ability to maintain a healthy self, they argue that they are also able to perpetuate and practice those symbols of Hawaiian culture that emphasize relationships with family and ancestors.

Healthy Differences: Views from On-Islanders

Most of the Native Hawaiians I spoke with on-island (63 percent) distinguish between being a healthy person and being a healthy Hawaiian. Healthy Hawaiian attributes include more than just taking care of the physical body. When asked, "Does it mean something different, from what you just described (a healthy person), to be a healthy Hawaiian?" responses included statements about how healthy Hawaiians maintain balance in life, knowledge about Hawaiian culture, and the ability to eat Hawaiian foods that come from Hawaiian land. For exam-ple, Ka'ala, a 39-year-old female social worker on Maui, emphasizes the impor-tance of Native Hawaiians maintaining balance in their lives:

> Hawaiians, I think, we have to have everything in balance, not just concentrate only on work, and not just concentrate only on play, but everything has to be equaled out and balanced. I guess, so in my mind, I'm imagining lōkahi where everything, our work, our play, our spirituality, our family, everything is balanced. And when one part of it gets off balance it kind of throws the whole individual off.

Ka'ala's statement is informative because of her emphasis on the word *lōkahi*. Lōkahi means more than just balance; it means having oneness, unity or har-mony with all the important aspects of life. These translations are mere glosses of what it really means to have lōkahi, as it references an experiential concept. As an experiential view of health it is the feeling of having all facets of our lives in harmony; one responsibility does not outweigh another responsibility. If, how-ever, lōkahi is taken as a functional view of health then it reflects an emphasis on moderation, not working too much or playing too much, because either situation results in poor productivity. In both interpretations, however, excess in any aspect of life can lead to illness.

Kupuna Lily, who is a kahuna lā'au lapa'au (a practitioner of Hawaiian medicine), turns our attention to another feature of Native Hawaiian health by focusing on the importance of eating Hawaiian foods and obtaining those foods from the land:

> Because the Hawaiians before were healthy and they ate their kind of food that they were brought up with. And they baked their food or they dried their food and, ah, they never had any fried food. They never used any sweetening thing. They used the sugar cane. If they had some kind of illness they have different herbs to use. They didn't drink coffee until the Americans brought the coffee over. They used to use herb teas. And afterward when they had the taste of coffee they start drinking coffee, which is not good actually for their bodies. Using oil for frying things, all the rich food. They never had those things. They lived off of the land, you know, whatever they plant, whatever they get from the river, from the ocean, that's what they live on.

For Kupuna Lily the transformation of diet plays the central role in defining Hawaiian health. She recognizes that Native Hawaiians are struggling to be healthy (as did most of my on-islander participants), yet she does not locate the source of the struggle only in the individual. Health is social, not individual. Food that is obtained from the land, rivers, and oceans of Hawai'i, food that Hawaiians were "brought up with," is the key to health. More explicitly, and yet similar to Ka'ala's view, there is a rejection of materials that represent foreign intrusions such as foods that are imported by Americans. Focusing on the foods that are consumed and how that food is obtained, produced or purchased begins to trace the ramifications of Native Hawaiian alienation from the land. Indeed, the majority of on-islanders pinpointed the transformation in foods consumed and how they were produced and acquired as the primary factor in poor health.

The meaning of being a healthy Hawaiian takes on other sociocultural attributes as well, such as the ability to speak the language, as Kaila, a 50-year-old nursing student states:

> I think to be a healthy Hawaiian means that you understand your culture. You know it's, this is the way we were raised when we were young, it wasn't a good thing to be Hawaiian. My grandparents spoke Hawaiian and we weren't allowed to speak Hawaiian. So we lost the language. My grandmother practiced the ancient religion but she didn't pass it on. And so we didn't learn the religion. So much was lost. I don't think I'm, I think there's a difference.—*So a healthy Hawaiian would be someone who's practicing those things?*—Uhm hmm. And understands what that means to be Hawaiian and how that's different from being a white, you know or an Anglo or whatever.

Kaila's quote illustrates her beliefs about the connection between a healthy body and a healthy society. Just as Native Hawaiian health has declined over the years, cultural knowledge has also been lost through the legal mechanisms instituted by colonists (e.g., schools) and the aging and passing of kūpuna who held on to that knowledge. The importance of regaining a self-conscious cultural identity, knowing how to think and speak as a Hawaiian, is key to being a healthy Hawaiian. Not only must one know what it means to be a Native Hawaiian and have pride in that identity, one must know that his or her identity is different from a "white" identity.

These women each express experiential facets of what it means to be a healthy Hawaiian. They all move beyond a mere attendance to the body's physical needs and turn our attention to a decolonization of knowledge and a relational basis of health. Significantly, this image is contrasted with transformations in the rearticulated Native Hawaiian way of life; lōkahi, eating Hawaiian food, and speaking Hawaiian versus an emphasis on work and production, consumption of food that was not from the island, speaking foreign languages, and believing in a foreign way of life. The contrast between Native Hawaiian and Western values is a key theme in the creation of exclusionary categories because the adoption of Western ways is viewed as the beginning of the decline of Hawaiian health. Opposition to the West creates a contrast and elaborates the relational features of power that provide a positioning for group identity, but more importantly it sets the framework for critiques of capitalist views of health.

Not all the people I spoke with in Hawai'i, regardless of age, sex, or income, thought that there was a difference between being a healthy person and a healthy Hawaiian. Further analysis of their responses, however, revealed that some differences do exist. It is important to note that of the 13 people who stated that there was no difference between being a healthy person and a healthy Hawaiian, 10 people later stated that eating Hawaiian foods would make Native Hawaiians healthier. Hawaiian foods were defined as fish, poi, and limu,[1] foods that come from the Hawaiian land and ocean. Despite their view that what is healthy for one human is healthy for all humans, they gave more importance to the purity and benefits of Hawaiian land and food, continuing the contrast between Native Hawaiians and foreigners as a basis for solidarity and a recognition of the inequalities embodied in access to specific foods.

Health is the Same for Everyone: Views from Off-Islanders

This same position was not as readily apparent for off-islanders. Indeed, when asked if there were any differences between what it means to be a healthy Hawaiian as opposed to being healthy in general, the majority of the off-island interviewees stated that there was no difference in meanings of health and that it meant the same thing to be a healthy human being as it did to be a healthy Hawaiian. The few who did point out that it meant something different to be a healthy Hawaiian had responses that were vaguely similar to the responses of those living on-island. Two people (17 percent) responded that having pride in being a Hawaiian, which also entailed being active in Hawaiian community service, was an important attribute of a healthy Hawaiian. Another responded that having good family relationships was important. Emphasizing family relationships draws on the knowledge that to be a healthy Hawaiian is more than just taking care of the individual body. It is not only that caring for others shows mutual obligations, but more importantly, a healthy body shows that you are part of the community, that others care for you. Finally a 25-year-old woman mentioned that Native Hawaiians eat too many saturated fats and processed sugars. Although her response is a misinterpretation of the question "does it mean something different to be a healthy Hawaiian?" it is revealing in that she believes that to be healthy in general was to eat a healthy diet (fruits, vegetables) and to get regular exercise. Taken with her statement that too many saturated fats and processed foods are consumed, we see a negation of the importance of access to resources and a statement about individual control over what is consumed.

For the most part, the off-islanders I interviewed regarded the health of Native Hawaiians in the negative sense and not as a consequence of unequal historical and political relationships with foreigners. The meanings of health and of healthy Hawaiians provided a contrast to the differences between them and their counterparts on-island. Unlike the on-islanders' abundant contrasts with the unhealthy practices that were brought to Hawai'i by foreigners, more often than not, the off-islanders compared their lifestyle habits (the things they do to maintain health) to family members living on-island. Typically the person I was speaking with would choose a cousin, sibling or other close relative who is obese or in such poor health that he or she cannot participate in the "healthy lifestyle" that the participant has chosen and views as the "correct" way of living. The reasons off-islanders gave for poor health varied, with explanations ranging from laziness, the cost of living in Hawai'i, to Hawaiian cultural attitudes in general. Although some of these reasons are the same as those given by on-islanders, their meaning is different. For example, the on-islanders emphasized lack of Native Hawaiian cultural values as the source of poor health, not that the cultural values caused poor health.

While discussing what it means to be healthy, Kimo told me about the activities he engages in to maintain his health, but then used the poor health of his sister to exemplify the need to exercise:

Of course you need to exercise.—*What kind of exercise?*—You really should do something regular. I've been dying to do something regular but it's so hard to find the time. I try not to take things too easy. Like I'm on the third floor office at work and I never take the elevator. I'm always running up and down the stairs all the time. I try to get out and walk, take the kids to the park. Do everything walking. And I know my sister is in such bad shape she wouldn't be able to do it and to me that's not healthy at all, so . . .

Later in our conversation we returned to the issue of health and activities Native Hawaiians can do to achieve better health; this time his wife (Wahine), who was also raised in Hawai'i, interjected:

Kimo: Don't eat too much kālua pig.

Wahine: Yeah get up and move around, they eating all that fatty stuff that pork thing.

Kimo: Well you can eat some of that stuff too if you go out and paddle a canoe often enough.

Wahine: Yeah, to get up and move around.

Kimo: I do have an awful lot of relatives that spend way too much time just sitting around the house. Probably just getting up and moving around is the best thing, and drink less beer. Some of the relatives are catching on to that. You saw how skinny Uncle looked last time we saw him. When he was about my age he was pretty fat.

Wahine: He gave up beer, he started exercising, and watching what he eats.

Kimo: Yeah he looks really good. He's about sixty now. Yeah he looks really good now.

Wahine: Your sister—that's scary, that's really scary.

Kimo: Yeah, she is definitely not healthy.

Wahine: She could lose 100 pounds and then she'd be okay.

Kimo: Ehh, I don't know if she has to lose that much, well actually, maybe.

Juliet: Is it her diet or everything?

Kimo: Yeah she doesn't exercise. When she comes here we like to go for walks with them after big meal. Especially after the holidays we have too much to eat. We go out for a walk. We live right next to the bike path here. So we'll go walk several miles. She can't keep up with us. She's younger than I am. Yeah and I'm yanking the boys, even when the boys were two, three years old, they'd walk miles with no problem and she just couldn't keep up. To me, that's frightening to be that unhealthy. But she won't listen to anybody. She's got a head of stone. That's the other thing. It's hard to tell Hawaiians what to do.

Health, for Kimo and his wife, is encapsulated in its dual aspects: eating right and exercising. In this conversation his sister has become the embodiment of what happens to you when you do not engage in these practices. Failure to do

these things further impairs your ability to engage in daily life, which my participants in California portrayed as relatively active. Furthermore, by referencing the
practices of an individual the social and historical factors that contextualize and
give rise to the poor health of Native Hawaiians is obscured. Poor health is the
sole responsibility of the individual who is further pathologized because of his
or her failure to achieve the health that in the individualized, neoliberal context
is available to all. Finally, in referencing Uncle as a relative who has "caught on"
to the need to eat well and exercise, Kimo and anyone who engages in "healthy"
behaviors is positioned as modern, one who is in the know, which is unlike his
stubborn sister who is stuck in the past, eating too much kālua pig and refusing
to exercise. Moreover, the attribute that is viewed as keeping the intrusion of
foreigners and foreign ideals in check, that is receiving health information and
care in Hawaiian contexts under the purview of Hawaiian elders is viewed as a
detriment, as revealed in the statement that "it's hard to tell Hawaiians what to
do." Health is made real by the image of the unhealthy Hawaiian.

The contrast between "modern" and "cultural" Native Hawaiians was further
explicated by Hoapili. Hoapili is 28 years old. She takes great pride in being a Native
Hawaiian and yet, until recently, she did not feel as intimately linked to Hawaiian
community activities in California. She has a few family members who still live in
Hawai'i whom she visits regularly. Her visions of health and modernity emphasized
eating properly and exercising, but these practices were indisputably separate from
representations of Native Hawaiian identity. The following is her response to the
question, "does it mean something different to be a healthy Hawaiian?"

> These kinds of things to me are the things, are more things to maintain a healthy
> body. Hawaiian is kind of who you are. It's not necessarily how you live, to me.
> It'd be like that with any race. If you focus too much on your ethnic background
> you're, you're losing a lot of the big picture. You're stereotyping yourself to fall into
> a particular category and to conform to a certain being. . . . It's, no you're a person,
> so therefore you should take care and maintain yourself as person. Not necessarily
> do a certain thing because you're Hawaiian. . . . I'm Hawaiian so I'm gonna eat you
> know the stereotypical foods they say Hawaiian people eat because I'm Hawaiian.
> No. You're a person you eat healthy, you need to exercise, you need to reduce your
> stress, . . . and last but not least yeah, by the way I'm Hawaiian. It's not gonna affect
> me because I may like certain foods so I may eat them because I like them. But I'm
> not gonna eat them just because I'm Hawaiian. I guess that's the way I look at it.
> But I wasn't raised real strict in any ethnic background. I'm just kinda who I am,
> and yeah, by the way yeah, I'm Hawaiian.

Health, for Hoapili, is again focused on the individual body. Lifestyle behaviors such as taking care of oneself and eating right have nothing to do with

ethnicity or the traditions of one's ancestors. The body is merely a body and does not represent the struggles of a people. The secularization of health and the creation of a generic body effectively wipe away any economic and political history, as well as the cultural battle to survive. Clearly Hoapili feels empowered to make choices about what she eats and how she exercises. It is at this point that economic differences between the on- and off-islanders are most clear. As individuals are empowered to make choices through higher income levels and education, there is often an increased reference to individual responsibility for health. As such, however, I would not argue that these differences are due solely to income. When Hoapili and Kimo's comments are compared to on-islanders whose average incomes are similar to the off-islanders in Orange County, the on-islanders had a greater recognition of colonial impacts and viewed culture as a strength that allows one to manage and resist structural barriers to health. It is the positive link to Native Hawaiian identity and values that help one to regain the health that was lost through colonial domination. In contrast, the use of health as a claim to cultural resources and Native Hawaiian identity was not a salient position for the transnational Native Hawaiians with whom I spoke. Issues pertaining to the struggle over health and land are not a prominent part of their daily context. Although class differences ease the path for individualizing health, location lessens the political and historical impacts that facilitate the perception that cultural values can be negative influences. Thus, Hoapili's case provides an interesting twist: through her ability to be a healthy person she also lays claim to her identity as a Hawaiian and through her individual survival she begins to build Hawaiian sensibilities. Indeed, shortly after our conversation she enrolled her daughter in a hula hālau and began to slowly build stronger ties with the off-islander community.

Sharing Identity and Knowledge

The revitalization of an alternative model of health for on-islanders highlights the subjugation of Native Hawaiian beliefs by colonialism, resistance by Hawaiians, and the ongoing struggle to renew Hawaiian identity through the conceptualization of what it means to be healthy. In contrast, off-islanders, while sharing knowledge of the domination of Native Hawaiians, do not struggle with their definition of what it means to be Hawaiian or of Hawaiian health on a daily basis. Their conceptualization of Native Hawaiian health is informed by images of poor health, stereotypes of Native Hawaiians and their lifestyles when they left the islands. Given the image of the unhealthy Hawaiian and of health as being under the control of the individual, off-islanders are not faced with a model of health that questions access to land and the ethnic socio-historical context as a rejection of a capitalist biomedical model that pervades their daily lives.

These contrasting contexts—rejection and reaffirmation of definition(s) of health—lead to specific expectations of what each group may think is needed to maintain health. Indeed, Blaisdell (1989) recognized the variation of Native Hawaiians' use of and belief in biomedical and Native Hawaiian medical practices. Reflecting the variation in views about health, the following section presents a comparison of the relative importance that each group (off-islanders and on-islanders) gave to practices of health. Cultural consensus and a visual representation using principal components analysis were used to measure the level of agreement within and between a sub-sample of each group on the ordering of practices needed to maintain health (Romney et al. 1986). The analysis suggests that, like Blaisdell (1989) and Hall (1994), there is a fluidity in the relative importance and meaning given to specific health practices that is influenced by place, but because of the ubiquity of biomedicine the differences are not exclusive to each place.

For a more systematic comparison of views regarding good health and maintaining good health, I chose to examine some of the data with formal cultural modeling methods. Understanding the role of cultural models not only gives us insight into current ways of thinking and interpreting behavior but also into its historical importance. Cultural models, as Holland notes:

> are significant because they channel experience of the present, inform anticipation of the future, and play an important role in the (re)construction of memories from the past. To the extent that these schemas [cultural models] arise from experiences interpreted according to a collective history and tradition, they are powerful cultural phenomena as well as psychological ones. (1992:68)

This definition of cultural models is reminiscent of identity and history issues highlighted by Hall (1994), Anderson (1991 [1983]), and Freidman (1994). These areas of study all emphasize the continuity of the present with the past, and that a collective history gives rise to representations in the present. Furthermore, collective history informs cultural models that are shared among people. The current and historical poor health of Native Hawaiians and its relationship to colonialism make the issue of health a rallying point around which to organize cultural models and revitalize a Native Hawaiian identity.

To accomplish the more formalized methods, I had a sub-sample of the people I spoke with freelist and then order (Romney, Weller and Batchelder 1986) those practices that best described what one must do to be healthy. First, early in the interview some participants were asked to discuss anything that, in their perception, was important to maintaining good health. I chose the top twelve items from their first freelist of important practices for maintaining good health for ranking (Table 4.2). These items were generated only from the on-island interviews[2] but are also similar to what the off-islanders mentioned, as noted in Table 4.1.

Participants were then asked to order the practices necessary for health from those that were the most important to those that were the least important for maintaining their health. I used cultural consensus analysis to test for the existence of a single cultural model that would reveal any underlying structures in the respondents' rank ordering of the health maintenance factors (Weller and Batchelder 1986; Romney, Batchelder and Weller 1987; Weller and Romney 1988).[3]

The ranking task reveals that the on-islanders, with a ratio between the first and second eigen values of 2.142 (a ratio of 3 to 1 is typically required), did not agree on the order of importance of items for health maintenance. In some cases, individuals thought that obtaining Hawaiian food, communing with the land, achieving lōkahi, and having good relationships were the most important for maintaining health. In other cases, having good relationships, having a positive attitude, getting enough exercise and eating a diet of fresh fruits and vegetables, and reducing stress were the keys to maintaining health. In contrast, the off-islanders do agree, with a consensus ratio of 4.019, on the order of importance of items for health maintenance. They typically rated having good relationships, having a positive attitude, exercise and eating fruits and vegetables, and reducing stress as among the most important practices for maintaining health.

A scaling routine is used to visually represent the level and pattern of agreement among Hawaiians (Figure 4.1). This was done by performing a principal components analysis to the agreement matrix (respondent-by-respondent correlation matrix on all the ranked items). The first two factors of the analysis are

Table 4.2. Ranking Items Important to Maintaining Good Health

Eating a good diet; fruits, vegetables
Eating a diet similar to our Hawaiian ancestors; fish, taro, limu, pōhole
Getting enough exercise
Communing with the land and ocean through farming or spiritually
Maintaining balance (lōkahi) between emotional, spiritual, and physical health
Having a positive attitude
Having a good spiritual life
Having focus in life
Regular salt water cleanse
Having good relationships with friends and family
Pride in who you are and in Hawaiian culture
Reducing stress

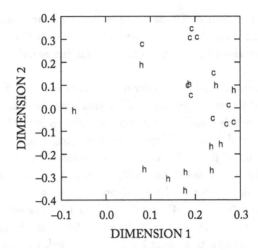

Figure 4.1. Visual representation of respondents' agreement on health maintenance items. The figure displays the spatial configuration of the health maintenance items obtained by plotting the first and second principal components. Each symbol represents the rankings of one respondent. The closer the symbols (h = Hawai'i respondents, c = California respondents) appear the more the respondents agreed about the ordering of the health maintenance items.

plotted; each symbol represents an individual respondent. Respondents represented as close together agree more than respondents that are farther apart.

Tracing the individuals vertically through this representation, we see a small grouping of off-islanders (c) at the top with an on-islander nearby (h). This grouping represents those individuals who thought that exercise and diet were among the most important factors for health. In the middle we see a grouping of both on- and off-islanders who represent those people who ordered having good relationships and having a positive attitude as the most important for health. Finally, we see a slightly diffuse grouping of on-islanders who rated lōkahi, eating Hawaiian foods, having good relationships, communing with the land, and having a positive attitude as among the most important for health. In this visual representation of individuals' responses to practices important for maintaining health we see a positioning that is responsive to both the dominant views of health and the struggle to revitalize an historically informed Native Hawaiian definition of health.

Observations in Hawai'i revealed that the meaning of health is in the process of being contested and reconfigured. As described in previous chapters, the social context in Hawai'i is one of heightened political awareness. The importance of viewing foreign intrusions as the source of poor health, and the image of the strong healthy ancestor are significant symbols in the revitalization of a Native Hawaiian identity and the critiquing of hegemonic discourses that are naturalized through health and biomedicine. More importantly, these symbols serve as motivators for action, which is a counter-hegemonic movement. As will be discussed further in Chapter 5, the call to life for the Native Hawaiian individual and social body is best achieved through the land, with all the food, spiritual, and economic resources that are imbued in the land. The relative significance of these symbols is being fought over, not just within the Native Hawaiian community but with the dominant Western health beliefs and values. The lack of consensus within the on-island group on the *ordering* of the items, which does not mean that they would not agree that the items are important, provides a picture of the struggle, of the ongoing reconfiguration of what it means to be healthy in Hawai'i. This is the key point: the Native Hawaiian model of health that I describe in Chapters 5 and 6 is an alternative model of health and identity, an alternative to the resident Western hegemony. Consensus analysis suggests that there are multiple models competing for hegemony; the use of health as a symbol for Native Hawaiian identity among on- and off-islanders is fluid, positioned between biomedicine, popular views, and the ancestors and contemporary Native Hawaiians.

The reason that the on-island group did not achieve consensus, I argue, is precisely the reason the off-island group did achieve consensus. There is no ongoing struggle in California or among the Hawaiian population to define what it means to be healthy. Their lives are bombarded with images of eating healthy and of people who exercise regularly. There is no significant land-based model of health that challenges the individual-responsibility lifestyle model that off-islanders are presented with. Thus, they agree on the order of importance for these health maintenance items, while at times incorporating the values of their homeland.

One unexpected outcome of the ordering of items from some of the off-island group was the top three items: having a positive attitude, having a good relationship with family and friends, and having a good spiritual life. Given their statements during my interviews I would have expected them to place eating right and exercising regularly as the top two items, followed by relationships, issues of land, and then living a life similar to the Hawaiian ancestors as the very last item of importance. These top three items, however, are both a part of popular discourse about living a quality life and are often associated with health discourse (Whorton 1988; Lupton 1997). Although these practices were not spontaneously mentioned in the interview, off-islanders are aware of their general importance to health both as Native Hawaiian and Western attitudes. The emphasis on these three practices might also represent the beginning of a shift in views about health for off-islanders. What is equally notable about the rank order of the off-islanders is that many of the themes that are deemed important in my interviews, such as the idea of lōkahi, eating a diet similar to the Hawaiian ancestors, and the importance of a relationship with the land for maintaining health were relatively unimportant for most of the off-islanders, as they were placed at the bottom of the rank order aggregate. At the time, there was no other model or discourse of health that was relevant or accessible enough in the daily lives of off-islanders. Consequently, off-islanders had no opportunities for a reconfiguring of beliefs about what it means to be healthy or to be a healthy Hawaiian.

Images of Health and Variation

Cultural consensus analysis proved to be a useful tool in further describing similarities and the differences between on-islanders and off-islanders. The lack of consensus on the ordering of the health maintenance items for on-islanders furthered the argument that there is currently a refutation of and a reconfiguring of health beliefs. In contrast, achieving consensus for the off-islanders reveals that despite their knowledge of Native Hawaiian struggles, evidence of that struggle to renegotiate their health beliefs, and by implication their identity, was not as readily apparent. The ways in which health becomes a position within these larger struggles, not only over politics but also for Native Hawaiians' livelihoods, varies by the ubiquity of biomedical discourses and the availability of Native Hawaiian discourses of health. This variation then is complicated by distance and represented in context.

The differences observed between off-islanders' and on-islanders' beliefs of health and identity speak very clearly to the issue of transnational identities. It is not merely that migrants attempt to re-create aspects of the lives they had in Hawai'i. Often, as is the case with off-islanders and issues of health, they choose practices that they view as promoting a "better" lifestyle than what they left behind. They define themselves in contrast to their relatives at home. Off-islanders are looking back to a point in time when Native Hawaiian health was viewed as a failure to abide by biomedical recommendations, and a time when Native Hawaiians were blamed for their social and economic conditions. Off-islanders' experience contextualizes a model of health that states that health is the responsibility of the individual. The representations, beliefs, and even daily practices that Native Hawaiians use to create their identity as off-islanders do not mirror the "home" they left behind; rather, their knowledge and practices are recontextualized, emerging from their experiences both at home and in California enmeshed in popular ideals of eating right, exercise, and having a positive attitude. Despite the lack of political struggle in their views of health, their experiences and practices in California perpetuate Hawaiian culture and identity through their existence. In contrast, on-islanders look back to a point in time where Native Hawaiians where strong and healthy. The image of what I call the "Healthy Ancestor" (Chapter 5) provides them both with a guide for achieving better health and a model that can challenge pervasive Western ideals. Despite the variations in views of health, we must not forget that these meanings have political and economic consequences for Native Hawaiian health, access to material and nonmaterial resources, and the embodiment of Hawaiian knowledge.

Endnotes

1. Limu is a type of seaweed.
2. Each health maintenance item was printed on a separate index card. I then asked respondents to put the cards in order, with the items most important to maintaining health at one end and those least important to maintaining health at the other end. This produced a rank order of the twelve health maintenance factors. When the task was completed, the respondents were asked what organizing principles they used to rank the items. Each rank order was aggregated by group, on-islanders and off-islanders, and then compared for similarities in the ordering of each item.
3. Cultural consensus analysis is a mathematical model that determines the degree of shared knowledge within groups and estimates the "culturally correct" answers according to the group interviewed. In other words, the "right answer" is determined by the interviewees' answers, not by a previously designed answer key. The analysis contains a measure known as "competence" that assesses the individual's expertise in relation to a set of culturally correct answers (the model) derived from a group of respondents' answers to questions concerning a specific domain of knowledge. I have chosen to use the term "agreement" in lieu of "competence" to express the quantitative relationship of the individual's expertise to the "culturally correct" answers, thus avoiding any confusion over the intended or unintended meaning of "competency." Cultural consensus analysis provides estimates of each individual's agreement and the average agreement level of the group. The analysis initially solves for individual estimates of agreement by factoring an agreement (correlation) matrix among informants. The ratio between the first and second eigen values determine whether a single factor solution exists, indicating a single, shared cultural belief system. Researchers in this field generally accept a ratio of 3 to 1, and all agreement scores falling between 0 and 1 (no negative agreement scores), as a minimum threshold for asserting that there is a single factor (cultural) solution. Cultural consensus analysis thus helps me determine respondents' agreement on the relative importance of the health maintenance factors, and on which health factors they disagree.

5

REMEMBERING ANCESTORS: FOOD AND LAND

Hawaiian health. I think it's good. They're, we're trying to go back to what we believed was helpful to us at that time. Like going back to the Hawaiian stuff is good. And we knew that at that time they, before them, before the white man came there was a whole lot of healthy people. You know, and never had all this kind sickness and stuff. So, if it was helpful for them at that time, I believe it would be helpful for us too. Provided that we can go back to that way. (Lani, a receptionist on Maui)

You get caught up in the rat race and the competition of what it's like to live in you know California, especially Orange County or Los Angeles, I think where it's really how you look. It's really how things are. And in Hawai'i . . . I think they're just happier with who they are. They don't have anything to prove. So yeah, I think it has a lot to do with us being in California is why it's so different. (Hoapili, an events planner in California)

In the overall sense of what it means to be a healthy Hawaiian, there were many similarities and differences between on- and off-islanders. These differences were often related to the context in which the islanders found themselves, reinforcing both the argument that we cannot afford to take definitions of health as "natural" (solely based on biological measures) and that we must continue to contextualize taken-for-granted categories that produce health inequalities. In this case, symbols such as "food" and "land" give meaning to an on-islander Native Hawaiian concept and contextualization of health and inequality. While we may assume that some foods are easily imported from Hawai'i, this is not always the case. Moreover, the actual land that is imbued with the mana from the gods is not portable either. One cannot transport Hawaiian land to California, and plants and foods, such as taro (kalo), breadfruit, and pōhole, while portable, are difficult to find. As such, health practices and their associated meanings as linked to food and land are recontextualized, and in different locales they may acquire different meanings. Does it mean the same thing to bathe in the ocean in Newport Beach, California, to tell your body that you are "home" after a long trip? Or, will the kalo that is grown in Irvine be imbued with the same mana as the kalo that is grown in the land where the Hawaiian ancestors were born? More importantly, as suggested in the previous chapter, in what ways are these meanings of health relevant for the daily lives of Native Hawaiians living in California? This chapter examines the importance of food and land for the maintenance and meaning of health, as well as their centrality in the process of place making. I argue that in remembering the ancestors through concepts of health, specifically land and food, there is a re-territorialization of both the Hawaiian Islands and a reconceptualization of the diasporic community. Calling our attention to these concepts and their use in a reconfiguration of identity in turn reveals an elaboration of the political economy of health for Native Hawaiians living on- and off-island.

Health and Land

As a symbol of a healthy Hawaiian identity, one key issue in the concept of "eating right" is the connection to land, the ancestors, and finally to the practice of acquiring and sharing food. For many of the on-islanders I spoke with, the importance of land for health was intimately integrated with food as a concept unto itself. In order to understand the importance of food, it is also necessary to understand the centrality of Hawaiian land as a health practice; that is, the importance of the ʻāina as a source of life and not just in the sense of providing food. For example, it is not unusual for many of us to consider a trip to the beach as a leisure activity. For Melelani, who is very self-conscious about her health and the foods she eats, a trip to the beach takes on more significance. Melelani knew that I was coming to talk with her about her views on health and how Native Hawaiians could be healthy again. When I arrived at her home one afternoon, she told me she wanted to take me to the beach, more specifically to the ocean, because that is where she goes to achieve lōkahi with the land, the ocean, and the ancestors, and ultimately to promote her health. "I brought you here," she told me, "so that you could see what we do as part of our health." It was not enough for her to talk about the importance of the ocean and land in her health practices, she wanted me experience the mana (divine power or life force) of the 'āina as it runs through the island and surrounding ocean. The embodiment of the 'āina for health includes origin stories and beliefs about the land's mana and its ability to heal, care, and provide for the people. Land is considered a deity in Native Hawaiian origin stories, which emphasizes the need to respect and care for it, to mālama'āina (Kame'eleihiwa 1992), in turn, the land will care for and feed the people. Making a spiritual connection regularly with the land and its power is an integral part of maintaining health.

The majority of people I spoke with on-island mentioned the importance of a connection to the land for health maintenance. Participants generally expressed two categories under which the relationship between land and health fall. The first category emphasizes access to land and people's ability to obtain things needed for good health. The second category emphasizes the importance of land for the restoration and maintenance of health, what I call land-based health. In raising issues of access and transformation, these categories call our attention to colonial and contemporary intrusions that make it difficult for or prevent Native Hawaiians as a group and as individuals from being healthy and highlight the complexities of a Hawaiian political economy of health.

Access to Land

In this section I examine two facets of the relationship between land and health and the creation of obstacles by capitalist development. The first category that reveals the relationship between land and health emphasizes Native Hawaiians' ability to access land and to obtain medicinals and traditional foods. Access to land has become an increasingly volatile issue. As capitalist production has expanded in the Hawaiian islands there has been less access to land for the Native Hawaiians (Trask 1993, Kelly 1997). More development and tourism, while seemingly good for the state economy, has led to protests[1] by Natives who desire greater access to the land and seek to prevent further encroachment onto undeveloped lands. Without access to land, Native Hawaiians lose an important resource for health maintenance. In acknowledgment of the constraining factors of capitalism, most of the participants (80 percent of the on-islanders) viewed a lack of access to land as an obstacle to health maintenance.

One issue that was at the forefront of many people's minds and provoked a multitude of protests from the Pele Defense League, sovereignty activists, local Hawaiians and environmentalists was the land transfers and development of the Wao Kele o Puna forest as a source of geothermal energy. Traditional healers, in particular, require access to forested areas to gather their medicinals. Located on the Big Island, access to Wao Kele o Puna forest was restricted when that area of land was transferred from the state[2] to a private owner, the Campbell Estate, in 1985. The land exchange cleared the way for geothermal development. Once Wao Kele o Puna became private property the Estate began restricting access to hunters and gatherers who had used that area for decades. Henry Auwae, a very well-known and respected kahuna lā'au lapa'au, established in his testimony for the court case against Campbell Estate that he had gathered plants and medicinals in the Wao Kele area since the 1930s. It was a place where kahuna lā'au lapa'au could gather medicines necessary for treatment of daily ailments as well as cancer and heart disease. Moreover, the medicinals from Wao Kele o Puna were stronger because of the environment (Kua 1994). Not only was the lack of access of concern to Henry Auwae, the effects of the geothermal drilling were "poisoning" the surrounding land, and during the development many trees and other vegetation were uprooted and torn down.[3] Henry Auwae's experience is an example of the widespread view that the lack of access to land and poisoning of land from outside, by non-Native parties, directly affects the ability of Native Hawaiians to practice Hawaiian modes of healing and health maintenance. From this perspective, continued development of Hawai'i in a manner that does not take into account the importance of the land in maintaining Hawaiian health will only exacerbate the health problem and limit cultural practices.

The lack of access to the land for medicinals and food is not only a problem for healers like Henry Auwae. Since mana, medicine, and health are found through food, pollution of gathering areas affects all who would choose to eat from the land. Nohea, a 49-year-old homemaker, also had Wao Kele o Puna on her mind when she commented:

> But, you know, progress came in and they cut all the plants down. See, on the Big Island, they're clearing all the land. And the Hawaiians are saying, "Wait don't do that, because the Hawaiian medicine is there, the 'awa." "[She is playing the role of a developer] But I gotta build the house, I got so much money invested in there. I got to take the plant down." And the Hawaiians are saying, "But wait let me take the plant out. Wait." "[Developer] No I don't have time to wait. Everyday is money." . . . And there goes the medicines. Even here on Maui, there goes the medicines. And even when you can find the medicine you have to make sure the area's not polluted so . . .

Nohea's role-play between the developers and the Native Hawaiians' plea to save the medicines is indicative of the relationship between Native Hawaiians and outsiders. The value of land has two very different meanings. For Native Hawaiians the value of land is medicinals and food, health, spirituality, and life. In contrast, the value of land for foreigners lies in the capitalist enterprise, that is, investments that make more money. Unfortunately, as evidenced by early contacts with foreign nations, the Māhele and the overthrow, this has long been the state of Native Hawaiian and foreigner relationships. The negative impact of development and pollution on access to Hawaiian land, food, and medicine extends to the supermarket shelves. Hawaiian foods that are produced and then sold to the markets also present problems of access. Kūpaʻa, a college student and single father of four, observes:

> Our Hawaiian diet has kinda like gotten out of hand for us as Hawaiians 'cause it's so expensive. You know try go to the market buy fish and it's all like, at times it's six to seven dollars a pound, and it gets up to 18 to 20 dollars a pound, depending on the season. And, you know, eating fish is healthy for you but buying a small little piece of it for 18 dollars is kinda outrageous. Trying to go out and find poi, which is a basic staple for us is really healthy, but try to go out to the shelf, you won't find it anymore. Now, when people want to shop for Hawaiian food, especially like for poi and stuff, they gotta know when the guys are delivering the poi, what store at what time. And when you usually go there, you see about maybe fifteen to twenty people standing there, waiting for the guy to open up the box. Our diet has pretty well gotten out of hand. Before we could go down beach and just harvest our own food. We've become so commercialized, and people out there before you and taking all the ʻopihi [type of shellfish], and picking all the limu [seaweed] and everything. And sometimes when it becomes so commercialized they're not thinking about tomorrow or next year. People pick limu and they just picking real fast and they uproot the whole plant. And so some places that used to have limu, it isn't there anymore. Because of development and stuff like that and the pollution in the ocean there a lot of places that used to have limu isn't there anymore.

The scarcity of poi in the stores and of limu in the ocean is a manifestation of the larger problem of access to Hawaiian food. Not many people have the time or resources to travel from store to store to find a "basic staple" of the Hawaiian diet. Furthermore, other foods to which Hawaiians typically had access are beyond the reach of the average Native Hawaiian's income. To eat a healthy Hawaiian diet of fish, poi, and limu is either very expensive or very time-consuming, and many Native Hawaiians are short on both money and time. Kūpaʻa gives us an excellent example of the barriers to accessing a Hawaiian diet from the Hawaiian land. The irony of the high cost of Hawaiian food is that these are the foods that can be the most abundant in the islands, and thus should be the easiest to find. Moreover, Kūpaʻa makes another link to the destructive forces of capitalism in highlighting the desire to have foods like limu and ʻopihi for the market without an accounting by producers and consumers for time or devastation to the environment. Development, pollution, and commercialization of land have effectively kept access to Hawaiian land and produce beyond the reach of the majority of Hawaiians.

Obstructing access to land through development, high food prices, and pollution is the same thing as obstructing the health and vitality of the people. Framed within a political economy that denies the connection between the use of land for social and physical health, the struggle for life and death in Hawaiʻi is obscured Kanaka maoli call for a recognition of land as both a political and an economic issue that is central to Native Hawaiian health and identity.

Land-based Health

The second category that emphasizes the importance of land for the restoration of health can be separated into two themes. The first theme deals with using land to increase spiritual and physical health; the second theme is centered on the use of the plants and land as medicinals.

Since land is imbued with mana (divine power), opportunities to interact with the land, whether through farming, bathing in the sea, or ingesting products grown from the land can be viewed as opportunities to interact with ke akua (gods). For example, Kūpaʻa told me a story of an event that exemplified the importance of land and spirituality when I asked him what things were important to maintaining Hawaiian health:

> Last week I had these Jehovah Witness come to my house and I didn't chase them away, but I sit down and talk with them. And then they already, from talking to me, they already knew that I had a faith. So they asked "Do you have a church?" "Oh yes, I have a church." Then after that they asked me "What church do you go?" So I told them Waipio Valley, that's what valley I go to. You know I do farming in there and that's my church. So I told them, it's spiritual there. I become aware of everything that ke akua, which we call god, created for us. And I feel more spiritual there than any other churches that I been in my life. I been in church where I see people falling asleep. I see churches where people sit down in there checking out their watch, what time it is, yeah. In Waipio there's no concept of time. I mean you don't feel tired or restless 'cause there's so much things there. And I find that's the best church that you know that I can think of . . . . So I think spirituality's really important.

For Kūpaʻa, the relationship of land and spirituality to health was so important that his response to my question about health was embedded in an example of spirituality. In addition, maintaining health means maintaining the health of the spirit through communing with the land, going to the valley and farming the land, and seeing all that ke akua created. Unlike the spatial and spiritual compartmentalization that a church building facilitates, Kūpaʻa is thinking of a more integrated form of health. His view of health does not represent the time constraints of clock watching or the limitations that a building enforces on the body. Rather, obtaining that balance between nature, spirit, and physicality is an achievement of lōkahi. Waipio Valley, on the Big Island, is an area that is increasingly being used by many people to start small gardens, mainly to grow kalo.

Similar to Melelani's story about swimming in the ocean as a part of experiencing health, another aspect of land-based health is interacting with the ocean. Hawaiians and other Polynesian societies use the ocean as a means of cleansing the body of any spiritual or physical impurities. For instance, Luomala states that:

> Hawaiians used salt water for sprinkling, to which they added turmeric and sometimes a sea rush or red ochre. Under a priest's direction, members of an entire Hawaiian community annually immersed themselves in the sea from midnight to dawn for purification, and afterward they feasted. Tahitians also had a comparable ritual, wherein all plunged into the "trackless ocean," "the supreme temple," to pray and wash off all spiritual and temporal crime and pollution. Individuals such as women after menstruation and childbirth, the sick, warriors or corpse-handlers had their taboo of defilement removed by immersion or sprinkling (1989:303).

Handy et al. (1934) also notes that, "The sea serves the same purpose [as fresh water] for both physical and psychic purification and restoration by sprinkling and bathing." It is not unusual for Hawaiians today to still use the purifying powers of the ocean. I was told about two primary uses of the ocean: the first is to cleanse and spiritually center the body, and the second is an internal cleansing of the body.

Melelani told me that whenever she arrives home after traveling, she always goes to the ocean within one day. She does this in order to center her mind and body, to let her body and the ocean know that she is home. She went on to say that if she forgets to go to the ocean she may get sick, or at the very least, she is unable to sleep well. For Melelani, the ocean has the power to tell her body that she is home, on the island where she was born, on the island where her ancestors were born. A prolonged disassociation with the land and ocean leads to poor health, a lack of lōkahi.

Another common practice is the salt water cleanse. Either purified ocean water or fresh water mixed with pa'akai (Hawaiian salt) is used as an internal cleaning of impurities in the body. People drink the salt water, which acts as a laxative, thus cleansing any internal impurities and restoring balance. The use of purgatives and enemas in the maintenance of Hawaiian health goes back to pre-contact Hawai'i (Handy et al. 1934; Kamakau [1866–1871] 1964). Traditional Hawaiian medicine seats emotions and thoughts in the na'au, the bowels. If people have bad thoughts or let their body, mind, and spirit get out of balance, then it will show up in their na'au. Thus, it is as necessary to cleanse the internal body as regularly as the external body to achieve lōkahi.

As the following examples will show, internal cleansing is a practice that had waned, but is experiencing a revival. Memories of cleansing are viewed by some as part of what Hawaiians did in the past. Several people I spoke with who no longer practice this type of cleansing did not view the failure to cleanse as a move towards a better way of life. Rather, they viewed cleansing as something they took for granted and stopped in order to go play with their friends, or to partake in the increasing number of "modern" activities that were being brought to the islands. One evening, Hoʻokena, a man in his mid-fifties, told me how, in preparation for enemas, his mother used to hang the bag and tubes in the bathroom. When he saw them there he always had a feeling of horror. He despised the times when his mother would call him in and say it was time for the cleansing. But now, he said, "I don't do that with my children, and they don't do it with their children. I always fought with my mother because I wanted to go off and play with my friends." The practice of cleansing is viewed not only as a part of health, but as something that previous generations practiced as both healing and preventive care but is now considered old-fashioned. The failure to regularly practice this type of health maintenance was viewed by the people I spoke with, and particularly Hoʻokena, as a loss of a part of Native Hawaiian culture and a move toward Western values.

While some people have stopped using enemas to cleanse internal impurities, it is not unusual for people to attend weekend or weeklong retreats where the main goal is to cleanse the body internally and regain pono through bathing in the ocean. There are often opportunities for both Hawaiians and visitors to enroll in cleansing seminars that are conducted by Hawaiian practitioners at hotels, offices, and even their own homes. During these retreats participants are given salt water cleanses, Hawaiian foods, lomi-lomi (Hawaiian massage), and are asked to discuss any troubles they may be having (a form of hoʻoponopono). The goal of the salt water cleanse is to allow your body, spirit, and mind to achieve lōkahi. As Pumehana, a lomi-lomi practitioner told me, people who do not cleanse at least twice a year are bound to get sick more often than people who do cleanse. She stated that it was a necessary part of one's health to rid the body of impurities that build up because of bad thoughts and bad foods.

Another example of the revival of salt water cleanses is their use after traveling. Alena, a lāʻau lapaʻau practitioner, mentioned that he always cleansed after traveling to remove all the impurities he had ingested from the different foods that he ate and drank. Moreover, it was a signal for his body that he was back home and could return to eating Hawaiian foods. Similarly, Melelani blames eating red meat and a failure to perform salt water cleanse as the cause of her most recent illness:

I find now that if I eat meat, I'll get sick. In fact this time I got sick I had eaten meat the night before it hit me. And I think if I had done the salt water cleanse, in retrospect, the very next morning, I probably would have resisted a lot better. The whole thing just came down on me.

The practice of cleansing with salt water is viewed not only as a healthy practice but also as something that rids people of foreign foods and values and ties people back to the land and puts their body back into balance with the islands. Interacting with and using food and medicinals from the 'āina, emphasize that the Hawaiian land is an ancestor that cares for your spiritual, cultural, and physical health. It is important to take note that these themes draw upon the broader knowledge of land as an ancestor, having mana, and the power to heal.

Somewhat surprisingly, in contrast to on-islanders, not one off-islander in California mentioned the importance of access to land to maintain health. There was no mention of the land or the ocean being used to restore health. When asked directly, however, 85 percent of the people who responded said that having access to land was important to having good health.[4] There was a certain amount of skepticism about how the land would be used. According to one woman, land is important to health "only if the land is going to be used to produce food to maintain healthy Hawaiians." Like on-islanders, this woman did not want to see the land further developed for capitalist gain.

For off-islanders, land was important primarily a source of food. One of the few comments I received that related the importance of land, health, and the ancestors was from Nu'uanu, a young woman who dances hula and wants to learn more about Hawaiian culture and her heritage as a Native Hawaiian. Nu'uanu stated:

> Well, I was taught that the old Hawaiians lived off the land, they grew their own food, and you know the taro and stuff. So that's why you see people now days fighting to get back the land, so that they can grow their own food and live like the old Hawaiians. But there's not a whole lot of people doing that, and even if they do get their land, like the Hawaiian Homestead land they usually don't grow food. Many people are just too Westernized now days.

While Nu'uanu knows about the lifestyles of the "old Hawaiians" and that it is something that many Hawaiians are fighting for today, she is skeptical that the outcome of more access to land will be the planting and growing of more Hawaiian food. By commenting on the "Westernization" of Hawaiians linked to the potential use or disuse of individual plots of land, she conflates "old Hawaiian" practices with capitalist values of individualism. There is an expectation that individuals should grow food on their private property rather than in communal gardens that facilitate social relationships and community health as in the ahupua'a system. The off-islanders I interviewed were more focused on the logistics of growing food. Kanoe also stated that if Hawaiians had access to land, they would need to learn how to grow food and be self-sufficient. Otherwise, in his opinion, the land would be just "another useless government handout." Off-islanders know of Hawaiian struggles and of the importance of land, but it is not knowledge that requires them to position themselves and their health in contrast to foreigners and their health. A difference between these groups however, is that land is a source of food production for economic gain and self-sufficiency and not primarily spiritual, a source of lōkahi, or as it is for on-islanders.

Healthy Food

Understandably, food and health are intertwined as simultaneously necessary for survival and as deadly when abused. In the United States, our everyday talk reveals our obsession with eating a healthy diet and even the morality of eating a healthy diet (Whorton 1988; Klein 1996; Leichter 1997; Kulick and Meneley 2005). There are a plethora of health magazines and fad and celebrity diets extolling the current health foods, saying that eating too much or eating too little food will kill us. We are told that high-fat diets increase the incidence of heart disease, cancer, and a multitude of other illnesses, and that a diet of fresh fruits and vegetables will make us lean and trim. As Crawford (1984, 1994) suggested, the food we eat becomes a statement of who we are, a window into our self, our body, and our mind. The degree to which we are able to control our relationship to food thus becomes a greater signifier of our national and cultural identity. The types of food one eats, the manner in which the food is prepared or even the amount of access to certain foods can be representations of class, geography or cultural capital (Bourdieu 1984; Bell and Valentine 1997). In saying that food consumption is solely a representation of individual or population identity and practices, the effects of access and the power relations imbued in defining "healthy" food are naturalized. Thus, an examination of the meaning of food provides another layer in the debate between Hawaiian and capitalist values. As the general meaning of health for both the on- and off-islanders alluded to, food plays a significant role in identifying the political and economic transformations that mark distinctions between Native Hawaiians and foreigners and between traditional and modern ways. The symbolic value of distinguishing types of food provides insight into on- and off-islanders remembrances of their distant and recent ancestors. In remembering ancestors the parallel categorizations and exclusions of *foreign* and *modern* are replayed in the meaning of food as are the constraints of a political economy of health that focuses on individual responsibility.

Food and Social Responsibility

It is not unusual that most Pacific societies mark food as central to creating and maintaining social relationships (Kahn 1986; Weiner 1988; Becker 1995). Sharing food with others shows one's ability to behave like kin. As one woman told me, "It's Hawaiian hospitality that we show you how much we care that we offer you something to eat right away." In Hawai'i it is customary to bring some food whenever you visit someone's home for more than a brief time. To arrive at someone's home empty-handed is considered shameful (Linnekin 1985). Sharing food engenders a sense of solidarity and reciprocity, an ability to care for each other that defines who belongs to the community. While reminiscing about the way things used to be before Native Hawaiians were taken from the land, Kalani, a 50-year-old man who works extensively with one of the sovereignty groups, states:

> I may be getting off the subject but, uh, see we're talking about the Hawaiian home-
> lands and they're [Westerners] taking all the good lands, but one of the reasons why
> the Hawaiians have suffered a lot was because they also took the Hawaiians away
> from the forest. So when the people used to come down from the forest and bring
> what they had in exchange for fish and whatever along the way you know, they just
> trade and take care of each other. So you had a system of sustenance because of the
> mutual cooperation and harmony between the people.

Here, Kalani is referring to the ahupua'a system, wherein the islands were divided into pie-shaped areas so that people who lived in the mountains could share and exchange food with those who lived by the ocean. Taking care of each other through the exchange of food is a highly valued part of building and maintaining a family and community. In the same vein, so is identify-ing who has been excluded from participating in the community, that is, the Europeans and Americans who removed Hawaiians from the land that enabled Hawaiians to care for themselves and those around them. Ikaika, a Hawaiian artisan, expressed similar sentiments: "Food in Hawaiian culture is a binding agreement. It is a spiritual and physical contract. For example, a baby lū'au is bonding the responsibility to the raising of the child." The importance of food for Hawaiians not only binds them to the land, it also binds them to each other, which makes their alienation from the land through Western capitalism a destructive act with far-reaching consequences in the creation and conduct of social relationships.

Sharing food with family and friends is one way that Hawaiians maintain their control of and pride in Hawaiian culture. In the quote that follows, Kūpa'a, describes his efforts to pass on Hawaiian culture to his children and younger generations. His efforts are not only seen in working the taro patches and in teaching his children to speak Hawaiian, but also in teaching them to obtain food in a traditional manner:

> I was working with juveniles, an alternative education program, we contracted with the State and we have 97 acres up in Wai'anae Valley. What we did was a restoration project, these are all ancient taro patches over four hundred years old. What we did is, you know, putting it back and making it work again. So I gained some experience in taro and I found some old Hawaiian fishing techniques like drag net and some other things in the ocean that are Hawaiian culture, culturally Hawaiian, and traditional. My son is encouraging. He goes fishing and stuff, you know. He brings home a meal about once a week, since he was . . . nine years old he's been fishing. Kind of reinforces in what he doing, it's not only fishing for sport, but comes home and feeds the family, that's good.

The restoration of taro (kalo) gardens is significant because kalo is not only the cornerstone of the Hawaiian diet, it is also a symbol of family, linked through the generations to their origins. In restoring the kalo gardens and finding traditional Hawaiian fishing techniques Kūpa'a creates an opportunity to practice the lifestyle of his ancestors and, more importantly, passes on to his son the importance of respect and caring for family and land. Using traditional Hawaiian tools to bring home food for the family is not merely something that is fun to do, a sport, it is also an action embodied with the tools and practices of the ancestors that ties them to Native Hawaiian history and culture. As such, it is a practice that reaffirms the ability to live on the land without the technology, knowledge, or development promoted by capitalist enterprises. Through the restoration, transmission, and practice of Hawaiian ways Kūpa'a and his son's actions are behaviors that are viewed as morally "good."

The extension of caring for family and community through sharing food was evident in the many restoration projects for ancient Hawaiian gardens (lo'i) and the creation of new gardens. On Maui and the Big Island I was told and read about numerous gardens for kalo and Hawaiian medicinals; many of these gardens were community projects. Individuals or organizations started the gardens to teach children how to grow kalo and give the community an additional form of subsistence. Local newspapers sometimes carried requests for people to come and work these gardens; Native Hawaiian youth are often actively recruited. It is an opportunity to remind them of their heritage through understanding the meaning of native plants and of how they are used for nutrition and medicinals. One organizer of a garden on Maui emphasized that the communal gardens are a very Hawaiian way of thinking about obtaining food. Indeed, I saw very few individual subsistence gardens in the homes I visited. The community gardens serve as an alternative place to gather food and as a symbol of sharing and caring for family and others. More importantly, the gardens provide a strong link to the practices of one's ancestors through work with the land.

More than "eating healthy," having a balanced diet of fish, fruits, and veg-etables, food and the obligations that are recognized through the acquisition and sharing of food are profound signifiers of belonging to past and present Native Hawaiian communities. The ability to maintain Native Hawaiian culture is, in part, seen in the ability to provide food, kalo, and fish for one other. The centrality of this meaning of food connects the symbols and practices of cultural identity to concepts of health. To be a healthy Hawaiian entails acquiring food from the land and ocean that your ancestors occupied and sharing that food with your community. It is clear that to be a "healthy Hawaiian" these ideals and the importance of the land do not only emerge out of a resistance to capitalist encounters; rather, they are an integral part of Hawaiian cultural knowledge and identity that are relevant for longevity and thus they demand that we attend to the system that produced the present-day inequalities and increased suffering among Native Hawaiians. The significant social land, food, and health associa-tions disrupt an emphasis on the individualized food-health dyad, thereby creat-ing the framework for debate and charting a future direction that is rooted in Hawaiian knowledge.

Differentiating Food

The symbolic value of food for community building is also seen in how it is used as a marker of difference in the production of health inequalities. Many of the on-islanders I spoke with mentioned a difference between Hawaiian food and Western or haole food and what it meant for their physical and political body. As Kupuna Leinā'ala stated,

we'd get everything off the land. And the only time I believe my parents really went to shop was for Western holidays, when they went to buy apples and oranges and stuff, buying the mainland foods. See we had our oranges, our own lemon. Then we started eating mainland stuff. And then, as the years go by World War II hap-pened along and everything changed and was never the same. And uhm, my health problem really started after I got married, the food was different from the kind that we had when I was a kid.

Unlike the communal gardening described above, for Kupuna Leinā'ala purchasing food is tied with the market and with shopping, which is a thoroughly capitalist mode of obtaining food. Types of food purchased and their location are further contrasted in that "Western holidays" are based on the mainland and not associated with Hawaiian cosmology, which is with the 'āina. From Kupuna Leina'ala's historical view, World War II is an important turning point in that the military build-up in Hawai'i during this time signified the growing political presence of the United States. The events of December 7, 1941 at Pearl Harbor, which was a violent statement of difference by yet another foreign nation, served to cement Hawai'i as belonging to the United States in the imaginary of American history. Hawai'i was no longer a territory; it was now headed toward statehood, and Native Hawaiians, despite their ongoing resistance, saw, as Kupuna Leinā'ala states, "everything changed and was never the same." As the political body shifted and the exclusion of Native Hawaiians from making decisions about their land and their livelihood continued, Kupuna Leinā'ala ties her worsening health to her increased intake not only of Western foods but also of Western values, which were brought on by her marriage. Whether her statement was conscious or not, there is an intriguing parallel to World War II and the health of the Native Hawaiian body politic, as Kupuna Leinā'ala was married to an American.

However, not all Western foods are seen as the cause of bad health. While talking about the eating habits of her family from Hana and their poor health, Mililani, an outspoken 38-year-old woman, makes distinctions between different kinds of healthy foods. Kalo and poi are considered healthy Hawaiian food, whereas fruits and vegetables are considered healthy haole food:

> It's just I don't eat any kind of food, that's why. If the family has diabetes, and hypertension and all those things, you have to stay away from high in fat. It says [diet books] you gotta eat a lot of vegetables, fruits, poi is good, taro is good, just staying more on the Hawaiian food. On the haole side stay on the vegetables and fruits.

Food takes on symbolic significance in distinguishing between Native Hawaiian and foreign identities. While there are numerous types of healthy foods, each represents affiliation with a group and includes the cultural memory that is embedded in the food. Health and the ability to promote health through a diet of good Hawaiian foods are part of a larger cultural model that emphasizes the purity of Native Hawaiian ways and their difference from other ways. This value and difference attributed to the role of food in health also lays the foundation for the importance of land in the revival of Native health.

Healthy Hawaiian Foods?

On-islanders contextualized food within political and family networks, shifting between food as signifying the purity of Native Hawaiian ways and the poor health that resulted from consuming Western-style foods. Off-islanders, in contrast, often spoke about how much of the Hawaiian diet was not good for you; pork, in particular. Hawaiian food was sometimes viewed as being either too salty, too fatty or both. Kupuna Nani, who has lived off-island for the last 25 years, recounted her memories of the unhealthy food Hawaiians ate when she was growing up:

> But Hawaiians are bad when it comes to dieting or, you know Hawaiians are bad because they eat a lot of fat, eat a lot of pork. I remember growing up maybe that's why we all have certain kind of illnesses because the pig, the kālua pig. You can't eat that without a little bit of fat on it. And uhm, they cook, they have Chinese cooking, Filipino cooking, but everything was centered around kālua pig that was the main dish. But that's where the illnesses are all, but they gotta watch.

It is important to notice that the other introduced foods, such as Chinese and Filipino cooking, are not viewed as the source of unhealthy food; rather, it is Hawaiian food that is the source of an unhealthy diet. This difference is in direct contrast to the on-islanders who viewed "traditional" Hawaiian food as healthy, and saw the introduction of haole food as the source of illness, ignoring the introduction of foods and cooking styles from other countries. On-islanders emphasize a different point in history, where Hawaiians were healthy and ate healthy foods such as fish and kalo that were abundant and easily accessible. In contrast, off-islanders look back to a time when they left the Islands and what Hawaiians were eating then: lots of fatty pork and salted food (salted to preserve food, because of the lack of refrigeration), which they then link to the poor health of Native Hawaiians. On-islanders emphasize the struggle to obtain what they *should be* eating, whereas off-islanders emphasize what they *were* eating.

Another difference that was apparent in my off-islander interviews was a distinction between local foods (foods that come from the many ethnic groups residing in Hawai'i) and, as they would say "Hawaiian, Hawaiian" food, that is food considered "traditionally" Hawaiian. For example, while Kimo was reminiscing about things he missed most about the islands, such as the ocean and family, he suddenly remembered food:

> Food, yeah, food, how could I forget food.—*What kinds of food?*—Well of course there's Hawaiian food, but uhm, just the local food back home. The fact that you can go to a plate lunch[5] place and get a decent lunch, better than fast food and real quick and it's cheap. And I don't know, it just has flavor you don't find here. All the

oriental foods, I mean you can get 'em here too, but they're just everywhere back there. All the fish, the fresh fish and it doesn't cost you an arm and a leg most of the time. It's just something everybody has.

For Kimo, Hawaiian food does not solely refer to "traditional" Hawaiian food. It also refers to all the other 'ono (delicious) foods introduced by other migrants over the years. Reminiscing about food in Hawai'i is not an unusual occurrence. For example, in many of the Native Hawaiian gatherings I attended in California, it was not uncommon to spend a significant amount of time talking about food and where to get food that is 'ono. However, what is considered "Hawaiian" food actually consists of the many different types of "local" food (Chinese, Korean, Filipino, and Japanese), that one can find in Hawai'i. When I asked people to give me an example of "Hawaiian" food, a common response was macaroni salad or kim chee. Unlike the on-island informants' views, Hawaiians in California define "Hawaiian" food as the myriad of local foods and dishes available in Hawai'i. Although not as 'ono as the local food in Hawai'i, it was definitely available in California. Off-islanders place greater emphasis on including other ethnic groups and foods or haole foods. While on-islanders certainly ate and enjoyed many of the local foods, there was a clear distinction between what was considered Hawaiian food and what was considered local food. Similar to my on-island conversations, off-islanders also talk about "eating healthy," which therefore becomes a category that includes different foods and different meanings. Drawing on the data from Chapter 4, it is not surprising that on the mainland, eating a healthy diet consists of fresh fruits and vegetables, and does not include eating foods from Hawai'i, like kalo and limu, implying a lack of shared cultural meaning with the on-islanders. The ability to eat healthy is not a symbol of struggle and is not a repudiation of Native Hawaiian identity. In other words, eating healthy has become more secularized for off-islanders. There are two potential reasons for this difference, both of which have to do with types of access to Hawaiian foods and fresh fruits and vegetables. The first reason is that eating a diet similar to that of the Native Hawaiian ancestors is not a key issue for off-islanders and has to do with the lack of access to island foods. Foods such as kalo, limu, poi, and pōhole are not readily available; they are not typically grown in California, nor are they easily imported. In contrast to the obstacles (such as developers, private property lines, and pollution) that prevent on-islanders from obtaining Hawaiian foods, Hawaiian foods are simply not a part of the locally available foods for off-islanders. While there is the option for people to go to one of the Asian stores that carry kalo, that takes time and involves making a concerted effort. Therefore, these foods are not thought of when considering how Hawaiians might maintain their health off-island. The second issue has to do with economics. Simply put, the price of fruits and vegetables in California is low in comparison to the prices of the same foods in Hawai'i. Recently a friend, Pi'iali'i, who lives in Hawai'i, told me of her last visit to California. She said:

> We were so excited when we saw the prices of onions and fresh fruits. We all ran into the market and bought a bunch of green onions, they were only 32 cents a bunch. We'd have to pay over a dollar here. We also bought some oranges and other fruits. Everything is so cheap in California.

Foods deemed to be healthy (fruits and vegetables) are relatively inexpensive compared to their price in Hawai'i. Consequently, accessing foods necessary for maintaining a healthy diet is both convenient and inexpensive. Similar to the issue of health insurance discussed in Chapter 3, the larger political economy of health in relation to food in California is ideologically and structurally supportive of hegemonic health practices, not Hawaiian health practices. This is not to say that all neighborhoods in California have equal access to nutritious foods—they do not (Frumkin 2005; Gordon-Larsen et al. 2006). In comparison to Hawai'i, however, "healthy" foods such as fruits and vegetables are easily accessible. Both these issues, the unavailability of Native Hawaiian foods and the lower prices of nutritious food in California, reveal the context-specific nature of defining what "eating healthy" means.

These two access factors work to hinder the consumption of a diet similar to that of the Native Hawaiian ancestors; "eating healthy" for off-islanders does not take on a meaning that could be used to reconstruct a shared vision of health and cultural identity and political struggle, which would position off-islanders as more similar to on-islanders. As Kanoe told me:

> The whole Native Hawaiian diet thing, and what's going on with the Wai'anae diet is passing them [Hawaiians in California] by. They don't know these things. When they think of eating Hawaiian foods they're thinking of manapua, rice, and other stuff that isn't really Hawaiian food.

The image of health achieved though eating a diet similar to the Hawaiian ancestors is not an effective representation of their struggles and thus has a different meaning in the everyday lives of off-islanders. Rather, their emphasis is on eating generically healthy foods, in the belief that what is healthy for one is healthy for all. Recontextualizing food for off-islanders thus reflects a Hawaiian subjectivity that suggests the primacy of "caring for the self." While this vision works as a discourse for survival and a perpetuation of the Hawaiian way of being, it shifts the focus back to the food/health dyad that makes individuals responsible and does not contest or attempt to reconfigure the inequalities produced within the mechanisms (food prices and access, insurance, access to health practitioners) that give rise to the current hegemonic view of health.

A Return to the Diet of Our Ancestors

There are multiple ways in which knowledge of nutrition gives legitimacy to hegemonic positions as well as contradicts those positions. A model of how Native Hawaiians can live and practice health through access to cultural knowledge, spirituality, food, and land is taken from pre-contact Hawaiians. In this view, the Hawaiians of old embody many aspects of the life that contemporary Hawaiians envision for themselves and their children. In terms of health, the hope for future generations is often seen in a return to a diet similar to that consumed by early Hawaiians. This discourse builds on both a romanticization of the health of ancestors and on current medical discourse concerning the need for a healthy, low-fat, balanced diet. Thus, a "traditional" diet is not only imbued with the strength of the ancestors, it is also legitimated in terms of contemporary scientific evidence. The symbol of the person I call the "Healthy Ancestor" provides a powerful metaphor not only for the purity of a Native Hawaiian lifestyle in the past, but also represents what it should be now and for future generations. Hawaiian ancestors are portrayed as strong, athletic, spiritual people who grew and harvested their own food (kalo, in particular) and most of all, they had unlimited access to the land and sea; they are the embodiment of all things "Hawaiian."

As noted earlier the Waiʻanae Diet Program is backed by knowledge that has been scientifically tested. This program produces an image of a Native Hawaiian nation as that of healthy people living off the land, eating a diet that was passed on to them through the generations, a diet that they must now struggle to regain.

Knowledge of the Healthy Ancestor is evident in the writings of academics and health officials. The notion of the Healthy Ancestor is also a part of how the Native Hawaiians I interviewed imagine their potential for good health in both lifestyle and body, for their past and their future. Sixty-nine percent of the on-islanders I interviewed described the Healthy Ancestor at least once in our conversations. This metaphor is made more poignant by contrasting the ancestors' lifestyles with contemporary problems such as the lack of access to land and Hawaiian foods; the plethora of processed foods, grocery stores, and fast food; and the generally poor health of Hawaiians.

In conjunction with shifts in diet, the lack of disease and germs is another major characteristic of the Healthy Ancestor. According to Melelani's recollections, ancient Hawaiians were able to live relatively germ-free and environmentally clean lives:

> I mean AIDS did not exist. That is, that's a twentieth century disease. Cancer if it's that old, I don't believe that it was that much in Hawai'i before, pre-contact. I don't, I, I just don't think so. If your lifestyle was clean, cleaner . . . can you imagine living and sustaining your life from the reef, from the mountains . . . . And that the stream is flowing, and that the taro is growing in the streams and the ōpae, and the hihiawai is growing and so you have your fresh water shrimp. You have the birds wherever you can get them and you eat them and you . . . you're eating the fruits and then, and then you have the reef, can you imagine? Catching a fish on the reef and eating right there? I mean, talk about eating fresh fish.

The purity of pre-contact life in Hawai'i is held in high esteem. The historical decimation of the Hawaiian population through disease and alienation from the land is held as the implicit marker of what foreigners have accomplished in the islands. This same marker, "pre-contact" also stands as an explicit example of the idealized life of the Healthy Hawaiian Ancestor.

Time and again, on-islanders acknowledged the health problems that they and their peers face. This acknowledgment, however, consistently drew on the coming of foreigners, the "white man," to historically position and explain the plight of on-islanders. To explain their current health problems, the contrast with the Healthy Ancestor provides a positive image of Hawaiian life and health. Moreover, the Healthy Ancestor is an image that contradicts scientific discourses as well as morbidity and mortality statistics that cast Native Hawaiians as naturally susceptible to poor health outcomes. Rather, Native Hawaiians are a strong and healthy people whose current health status is reflective of social inequalities that can be amended.

The pervasiveness of the Healthy Ancestor is apparent in many interviews regardless of the speaker's tendency to identify with Native Hawaiian practices or causes. Sometimes references to the Healthy Ancestor would simply be recommendations to return to traditional Hawaiian ways. For example, Ipo, a 28-year-old energetic man, had very little to say about practicing Hawaiian culture or gaining access to land. Even though differentiating himself as a Hawaiian was not very important to him, he saw the value of a Hawaiian diet in maintaining health:

> Well, I wasn't living in the ancient ages. But how I heard and how we study here and everything what they used to eat and when the Western society came into Hawai'i. The Western society changed, like you know maybe now people get lazy to cook, so McDonalds. McDonalds is all that oil and stuff, so it's that's how I

think. Because when we do the Waiʻanae diet, people can get off insulin, can get all these things just from the nutrients and all these things just from the nutrients and things, they, they go back to the ancient ways.

The perceived health and lifestyles of ancient Hawaiians cannot be overestimated when considering the contemporary revitalization efforts. The historical connection does not end with the ancestors' lifestyle as a prescription for good health. As stated earlier by Kūpaʻa, to be a healthy Hawaiian one must have access to land.

The Healthy Ancestor is held up as the example of what life should be like for Hawaiians, and what it would be like if they could get back their land. The loss of land combined with the findings from the Waiʻanae Diet Program (1993) and the Molokaʻi Heart and Diet Study (Curb et al. 1991) further bolster the argument that Native Hawaiian alienation from the land is associated with poor health outcomes. As Kuʻumeaaloha Gomes, a native Hawaiian scholar and activist states:

In talking about health, you must talk about food, so you must talk loʻi (gardens)— and so you've got to talk golf courses, and so you've got to talk foreign investments. . . . It's not just a "cultural perspective"; it's who we are as a people, as political and socioeconomic thinkers. (Quoted from Scheder 1993:29)

For Gomes, achieving health means growing more kalo and stopping the development of more golf courses that consume resources that can be used to achieve health. Acquiring a health status similar to that of the Healthy Ancestor is inherently a political matter. It reveals the Hawaiians' historical struggles with foreigners over land, to which food, ideologies, and life are intimately tied. Similarly, Dr. Kekuni Blaisdell states, "It is essential that adequate resources be provided to produce proper foods: taro, sweet potato and fish. But gardens are displaced by golf courses, and there is a constant struggle for adequate water (quoted from Scheder 1993:29)." Gomes and Blaisdell are among many in the health field who are calling for a critical look at interventions designed to "improve" the health of Hawaiians that only look at individual-level behaviors. They are calling for an active stance that seeks to better health by improving access to Hawaiian food and land. Based on decades of research and experience Shintani, Aluli, Gomes, and others agree that a diet similar to that of the early ancestors will improve the health of Native Hawaiians. More importantly, these authors promote the argument that to achieve that health Native Hawaiians must have land to practice the lifestyle of their ancestors. The combined knowledge of nutrition research, links to a shared pre-contact history, the integration of the Healthy Ancestor into the discourse of everyday life, and the recognition of the inequities produced by the current system of health have put into action the elements necessary for a powerful counter-hegemonic movement aimed at transforming Native Hawaiian health.

Locating the Healthy Ancestor

Like many aspects of Native Hawaiian health, the image of the Healthy Ancestor is contested among Hawaiians themselves, as the analysis in Chapter 4 suggested. In contrast to using contact with the West as the principal event that triggered the reign of Hawaiian poor health as the on-islanders did, off-island interviewees rarely mentioned, implicitly or explicitly, any negative health effects or long-term effects of contact with the West. Kimo, who is very active in one of the Hawaiian civic clubs and travels regularly to Hawai'i for weddings, funerals, and other family events, gave the only response stating that any illness was caused by contact with the West:

> My kids both have allergies and I do too. It comes down . . . I think actually my mother's side. She was almost pure Hawaiian. She was seven-eighths Hawaiian. And that one eighth, that means she had one great grandfather who was not Hawaiian, and that's where the name comes from too, Smith [pseudonym]. He was an Englishman. He was not the oldest who would inherit the land. So he went to seek his adventure in the world. Ended up in Hawai'i. Married a Hawaiian. So now there's a whole family in Kona named "Smith," because of that one Englishman. And I think he gave us the asthma [laughs].

In comparison to the characterization that most poor health dates from the introduction of Western ways of life, capitalism, food, and germs by on-islanders, this introduction of asthma into the family line appears rather benign. The West as the source of illness is not a salient theme for off-islanders. I did not get the impression that they were reluctant to place that kind of blame on the Europeans and Americans who came into contact with early Kanaka Maoli or that the exclusionary category was even necessary in the construction of their cultural identities as healthy Hawaiians. The context for off-islanders does not require them to represent struggles with the West in the same way that on-islanders represent and engage in the debate over land and health.

When talking about the health of earlier generations most off-islanders seemed to focus on the poor diet of Native Hawaiians. When comparing the health of Hawaiians today with the health of earlier generations, Kupuna Nani stated:

> I think today should be better. Because now days, I never heard don't eat fat because cholesterol. Don't eat this because heart attack, don't eat that. But now there are

studies on it so the people are aware if they're eating that kind of stuff it's their own fault. In our days we were not told. Maybe somebody knew, but it wasn't out like now. The papers and magazines they tell you. Health magazines you know. Before you eat what you wanted and nobody told us. And they died younger. But they were happy because they ate everything they wanted. But now days you can but you know what's gonna happen because they tell you.

Kupuna Nani's attention to the health studies and popularity of health trends towards eating less fat and lower-cholesterol foods guides her reinterpretation of the health, or rather the poor health, of previous generations of Hawaiians. Furthermore, the new, modern knowledge that is available locates the blame in the individual "if they're eating that kind of stuff it's their own fault." This position on health not only fits with Crawford's 1984 analysis of middle-class American views of health as a matter of self-control, it also reflects the increasingly neo-liberal views of health that emphasize individual empowerment through the freedom to make good choices. Unfortunately the emphasis on self-control and individual choice is cast against a historical and sociopolitical context that provides better options for those who can afford more choices. For Kupuna Nani, the context of better knowledge about health processes gives her an explanatory model for the early death of Native Hawaiians and the poor health of the Hawaiian population. In attending to the scientific and individualized knowledge, the critique on inequality in Hawai'i is obscured and ancestors are not called upon to redefine health.

After a significant amount of probing, Kimo was the only interviewee who brought up the image of the healthy Hawaiian ancestor:

—*What about even further back in Hawaiian society?*—Hmm . . . hard to tell. They seemed to be pretty healthy. The Hawaiian race as a whole got bigger and stronger through the generations. Modern analysis has shown that taro is about the most perfect food for humans. If you could invent the perfect food it would probably be taro. It's very nutritious and it's low in fat and uh, and the old Hawaiians did get a lot of exercise. Even their entertainment seemed to be more physical. They had kōnane [type of checkers game] and things that weren't very physical. But the other things, you know hunting, and spear throwing, and canoe paddling and surfing. Those will keep you in shape.

The emphasis is again on a low-fat diet and getting enough exercise. Living an active life, which is what the ancestors were able to do, is the key to being healthy. Like the images of the healthy Hawaiian provided by the Wai'anae Diet and Native Hawaiian health studies on-island, these statements are based on current scientific knowledge about diet and nutrition to support the understanding of what is good for a healthy body. These quotes, however, lack the attention paid to the Healthy Ancestor that was apparent in the on-islander discussions. More importantly, they do not carry any motivating force such as a moral agenda that says that living like our ancestors will make us healthier.

While both on and off-islanders draw on contemporary views of how to achieve health, from the Wai'anae diet to popular health books and magazines, in one case health is firmly located in the practices of the past whereas the other is based in the practices of a generic body, one that has equal access to healthy foods and activity. These different visions for health reflect debates over whether health is the responsibility of the individual or of society. For on-islanders the issue of land, health, culture, and sovereignty are intertwined social responsibilities. For off-islanders health is abstracted from its context and the sole responsibility of the individual is to make sure they eat the right (low-fat) foods and incorporate exercise into their daily routines so that their physical body will remain healthy.

Meanings, Models, and Portable Symbols

The off-islanders I spoke with subscribe to a popular model of health that focuses on the individual. If you eat right and exercise you will live a healthy life; no matter who you are or where you come from, good health is attainable for all. The common critique of lifestyle behaviors as the cause of poor health is that it overlooks the context in which the poor health occurs and it blames the victim for circumstances that are the cause of policies that benefit those in power. Focusing on individual behaviors allows us to ignore the context in which poor health develops.

This attitude of placing blame on the individual for poor health becomes controversial when Native Hawaiians return home. In my many conversations I would hear people (Hawaiians and non-Hawaiians) say "Hawaiians are stubborn," or "you can't tell them anything." The emphasis on changing lifestyle behaviors for on-islanders is often interpreted as another intrusion by haoles or, as discussed in Chapter 2, is seen as an extension of a colonial agenda. A few of the people I spoke with in Hawai'i referred to themselves as "transplants," individuals who just returned "home" after living on the mainland. When they suggested differences in lifestyle that are prevalent on the mainland, such as drinking less alcohol, not smoking cigarettes, and eating less food, they were told not to bring their 'ōpala (trash) to the islands. This attitude suggests that what is known to be a healthy lifestyle on the mainland is viewed as an intrusion of haole ways and is contradictory to Hawaiian views. On-islanders are no longer willing to take the sole blame for poor health and are prepared and willing to establish the relationship between the decline in health and colonization; they also point out the contradictions inherent in blaming individuals for their poor health. The health crisis that was readily apparent in Hawai'i was not part of the discourse on the health of off-islanders. The economic and political context in California removed Hawaiians living here both geographically and culturally from the issue of health as part of their political and cultural identity. Health inequalities do not produce salient symbols for the re-creation of a Hawaiian identity in California. Thus, to be healthy it is not critical to have a connection to the land, have access to the land or obtain mana from the land. Hawaiian land is not portable and therefore is not reflected as necessary to daily health practices for off-islanders. While the Healthy Ancestor may have some meaning as a symbol, it is not significant as an aspect of health in building a shared history or in imagining the Hawaiian nation.

However, there are many portable symbols used by off-islanders to create a sense of community and to recontextualize their "Hawaiianness." For example, participating in hula hālau, hula competitions, annual festivals, and returning home to share and be with family are potent symbols for off-islanders. Hula is one of the more prominent activities off-islanders use to show respect for their ancestors and to maintain family ties. Attending the many Pacific Islander festivals allows Hawaiians and other islanders to gather and reminisce about island life, to sing songs, and to eat "local" foods. Hawaiian off-islanders work very hard to promote and attend Hawaiian cultural events. Recall that the Hawaiian club, Nā Mamo, organizes one of the largest hula competitions outside of the islands. Other Hawaiian clubs are active in sponsoring Hawaiian language classes and weekend retreats that focus on teaching families Hawaiian values. The majority of the off-islanders I spoke with made multiple annual visits to see family in Hawai'i. In this way, Hawaiians in California are perpetuating Hawaiian culture, respect, and remembrance of their ancestors. In leaving the unhealthy habits that were prevalent on-island they have become "healthy Hawaiians."

Hawaiians in California also have an awareness of the economic struggles that their relatives have in the islands. Half the people I interviewed in California mentioned the high prices of foods and the low wages that Native Hawaiians receive. The economic and political context in Hawai'i today is not similar to the context in California. The Native Hawaiians I spoke with in California make a decent living. They have college degrees and well-paying jobs, which are the key reasons why most of them left the islands for California. They do not struggle to make ends meet to the same degree as many of their counterparts in Hawai'i. They do not have to pay exorbitant prices for fresh foods, or foods that are grown on the land that is right in front of them. Hawaiian land is not a symbol that is portable in that one cannot take acres of land from Hawai'i to California and imbue it with the same meanings and energy that it had at home. This position is evident in the lyrics from Mark Hoʻomalu Kealiʻi that was used at the opening of the book. Native Hawaiian bodies off-island become the living ʻāina that one must mālama. Therefore, there is no struggle over the meaning or access to Hawaiian land. The context in which off-islanders live requires them to position themselves differently than their counterparts in Hawaiʻi.

While many Hawaiians in California maintain their Hawaiian identity through participation in clubs, festivals, language courses, and hula events, their lifestyle calls for a different interpretation of health and what it means to be healthy. The circumstances in Hawaiʻi that enable land, history, health, and identity to be intertwined are weakened for Hawaiians in California and the call to life does not entail Hawaiians contesting the pervasive Western definitions of health.

The Call to Life: Reconfiguring Health and Identity

For the on-islanders I interviewed, an emerging cultural model of health offers an opportunity to contest and reconfigure the currently hegemonic models of health. On the surface the model appears to be a replica of popular health issues such as eating right and getting enough exercise. A more in-depth analysis, however, reveals that eating right has a meaning system attached to it that touches the roots of Hawaiian cosmology. The maintenance of a healthy Hawaiian body means attaining lōkahi with your spirit, your culture, and the land. Hawaiian foods come from Hawaiian land and sea, are imbued with mana, and have the power to heal. This ideal lifestyle is embodied in the memories of the Healthy Ancestor, a shared memory that can offer new visions and expectations of the future. The pre-contact Hawaiian ancestor is an image of beauty, strength, and health. Living off the land by farming, hunting, fishing, sharing food, and caring for each other and the land will return health to the Native Hawaiian population. Health concerns throw into relief the material and cultural dispossession of a colonized people. As Native Hawaiians engage in identity politics, land becomes a rallying cry for life itself. The Hawaiian ancestor represents an ideal healthy lifestyle and identity and the knowledge base for a counter-hegemonic movement. It is in the search for health that Hawaiians find the Healthy Ancestor, kāhea ola—the call to life.

This growing call to life sets the stage for turmoil, for a reconfiguration of what it means to be healthy, to be Native Hawaiian. It is a challenge to reintroduce issues of land, "traditional" foods, and plants into a conceptualization of what it means to be a "healthy Hawaiian." Western culture rolled over the islands like a tsunami, oppressing, repressing, and silencing Hawaiian culture. The importance of the relationship between the elements—land, history, and health—challenges Western ideals of health as an individual's responsibility. The issue of Native Hawaiian health is a joint concern of biomedical practitioners, public health officials, Native Hawaiian scholars, promoters of a Hawaiian renaissance, promoters of sovereignty and, most importantly, of average Native Hawaiians. While they all agree that achieving good health is important, they do not agree on how best to achieve it. What does this mean for Native Hawaiians' everyday lives, their health experiences, and their identity? Hawaiians have presented once again an alternative model of health, one that is meaningful because it emerged out of their pre-contact experiences and engaged their colonial and neocolonial struggles. It is hard to tell whether this Native Hawaiian model will become the hegemonic way of thinking about health. What we do know is that Western ideals will no longer reign supreme and uncontested as the best way to achieve health or the best way to live as a Native Hawaiian.

Endnotes

1. Just looking at the 1990s there were numerous protests on issues ranging from the geothermal development in Wao Kele O Puna Valley; the Anti-Annexation March, which focused on the illegal overthrow of the Hawaiian monarchy and annexation by the United States in 1898; Protect Kahoʻoʻlawe, which worked toward stopping military bombing of the island and returned the land to the State; and homelessness. All these issues are linked to efforts to regain Hawaiian sovereignty.
2. The state was assigned as a trustee for the 1.4 million acres of "ceded" crown lands at the time of Statehood. Recall that the crown lands were "ceded" when the islands were annexed by the United States. This land has been leased out for education, airports, and military uses. Other areas have been set aside for Native Hawaiian Homelands and National Park Reserves. Unfortunately, much of the prime land, which is usable agricultural acreage and ocean front areas, has been exchanged with private owners for tracts of land that were not usable for living or subsistence (Trask 1993; Office of Hawaiian Affairs 2009).
3. See Pele's Appeal for documentation of the land that was razed and the plants that were destroyed in preparation for the development of Wao Kele O Puna. In 1994 the geothermal project was abandoned making way for the sale of the land in 2001. With significant funding from the USDA Forest Legacy Program, OHA was able to purchase the property in 2006 preserving the area for cultural and conservation purposes.
4. Four of seventeen had no response to the question and two said that land was not important at all to the maintenance of health.
5. Plate lunch typically consist of fish or chicken, rice, and macaroni salad.

6

CONSTITUTING THE HAWAIIAN BODY: RESISTING AND REINTERPRETING HEALTH AND CONTROL

During the mid-1990s I often attended the Annual Ho'olaule'a Hawaiian Festival. One year, well over 5000 families and individuals had chosen to spend the weekend celebrating Hawaiian culture at Alondra Park, California. A variety of events throughout the day included hula performances, lei making, music, various vendors, and some local artisans. The air was filled with ono (delicious) aromas of local Hawaiian foods. It was a beautiful day to be out in southern California. While I was enjoying the sights and sounds of all the festivities, Noelani, an off-island woman I had known for over four years, made a comment about the body size of Hawaiians, which forced me to think about the complicated views of the body as a representation of health and of the revitalization of health. We wandered among the many booths, stopping at a T-shirt vendor, and I was struck by how many were already "sold out," as indicated by various stickers. Noticing that the majority of the sold-out sizes were XXL, Noelani laughingly remarked, "Oh, that happens a lot. You know Hawaiians! They're big people!"

Among Pacific Islanders, "body size" is an important and often the most significant descriptor in characterizing social relationships and health. Similar to the variations in emphasis on land and food as key components to health, political and economic influences were reflected in the meaning of body size. On- and off-islanders used body size to comment on issues of control, place, and ultimately on individual and social health. For off-islanders, however, large bodies were more problematic than for on-islanders. It is not that any of the

off-islanders were physically smaller, or even considered themselves smaller, in
size when compared to on-islanders. In fact, in my own estimation, I would say
that all the people I spoke with, both on- and off-island, ranged in body size to
the same degree; some were quite large, some were average in size, and a few
were thin and petite. Given this observation, I began to ponder the significance
of body size, specifically the divergent views regarding the body and its relationship to health.

In this chapter I argue that the meaning of the body and health is contested in
ways that reflect the struggle between the desires of capitalism's productive body
and a body that reflects the historical and cultural conflicts of Native Hawaiians
and their efforts to regain political and economic sovereignty. Health, like the
body and land, are taken to be "natural," that is, their composition, functioning,
and existence are often presumed to be the essential and untainted components
of life. In other words, the land-body connection is remade in a historical-cultural
reading of the body, while simultaneously being linked and at times de-linked
from place and nature through capitalist readings of the body. Linking processes
of identity and material flows with body, health, and land remind us that the
body, like health, can never be considered "natural" (Foucault 1979; Bordo 1993).
Bodies, and thus body size, are created, represented, and interpreted through
cultural and material practices, and are subject to technologies of power associated with medical and popular health discourses. The interrogation of large bodies provides an opportunity to offer alternative versions of representations that
contest capitalist interpretations of the body and that emphasize the agency of
Native Hawaiians to rewrite the meanings associated with both a large Hawaiian
body and a fit Hawaiian body. The differences between on- and off-islanders'
definition of Native Hawaiian health as part of a revitalization movement is
reflected in struggles over the representation and meaning of the body. In this
chapter I provide examples of various representations and meanings of Hawaiian
bodies, highlighting the need to attend to the socio-historical, political, and economic contexts. More importantly, however, I discuss how the flexibility of the
body presents an opportunity for a counter-hegemonic movement to take on the
hegemonic discourses of health and imbue the body with Hawaiian meanings.
The representations of the bodies that I use in this chapter are a combination
of descriptions from interviews with on- and off-islanders in conjunction with
popular representations and interpretations of Hawaiian bodies. Although there
is a difference between on- and off-islanders' explanations for why people may
have large bodies, they both note the associated problems of such bodies, such
as decreased life spans, and argue that action must be taken to stem the tide
of poor health caused by obesity. Previous chapters have provided contextual
and economic explanations for the differences between these two groups. This

chapter seeks to use the body, one of the most "natural" and malleable symbols, to examine the potentials and constraints of a Hawaiian view of health.

Studies of the body often take the perspective that the body is an object, a representation, from which identities are read (Foucault 1979; Bordo 1993; Lock 1993). When bodies migrate, they carry the cultural knowledge of the homeland with them, as suggested by the lyrics of Hoʻomalu I cite at the opening of this book. Unlike land, which is not portable, memories, experiences, and bodies can be transported, thereby being caught up in the cultural flows of migration and globalization. The body is one of the more salient and tangible symbols of health (Benson 1997:123). This connection is, in part, due to the biological basis of the body that facilitates the ease with which cultural meanings and political and economic forces become naturalized, being viewed as inherent in healthy and unhealthy bodies. As Foucault (1979) and Crawford (1994) argue, medical discourses gain power over the body through naturalization as it is linked to Enlightenment, egalitarian notions that health is the presumed natural disposition of the body and that health is equally available to everyone. Bodies that do not maintain the health that nature has given them are failed bodies and "unhealthy others" (bodies that are not disciplined in the knowledge of health nor values of capitalist productivity) (e.g., Bordo 1993; Crawford 1984, 1994). This taken-for-granted view of the body creates identities that simultaneously suggest racial categories (unhealthy populations) as well as individual control—the dual meaning suggested by Noelani's comment about XXL T-shirts selling out so quickly. Scholars have long argued that representations of poor health are often used as a characteristic of race by colonial regimes (King 1987; Comaroff 1993, 2007; Anderson 2006). That ill health and obesity strike the poor and disenfranchised ethnic groups at higher rates (Flegal et al. 2002; Drewnowski and Specter 2004) and that those findings are subsequently used to support arguments that naturalize race and unhealthiness is an extension of historical relations and a creation of "others" (Said 1978; Lee 2008; Heurtin Roberts 2008).

It has long been noted that large bodies have been valued differently across time and societies (Garine and Pollock 1995; LeBesco 2004; Kulick and Meneley 2005). Currently, numerous studies show that the body, particularly in the Pacific, is a symbolic representation of strong social relations (Becker 1995; Cassidy 1991; Nichter 1991). Large bodies indicate that people care for you by sharing food and ensuring that you are well fed. In contrast, thin bodies indicate weak social ties, that no one cares for you (Becker 1995; Pollock 1995). For example, while working with Tongans in northern California, I was often asked why I was so skinny. Was I not being fed or did I exercise too much (these questions were not to be taken as compliments)? Despite these alternative meanings of body size, the image and statistics that cause researchers and the lay population alike to focus on the large body are medicalized, hinging on a representation of pathology. When a body is large or at the high end of the Body Mass Index (BMI), even though we are been told to account for larger bone structures like those of Pacific Islanders, such a body is assumed to be at risk for disease. Indeed, there is an abundance of social and medical work on the obese body, as well as the anorexic body, both representing opposite ends of control over food consumption, and both of which are deemed unhealthy. Medical discourses constitute a significant source of framing for the "unhealthy" fat body. Considering the high rates of heart disease, cancer, diabetes, and hypertension (diseases associated with obesity) among Native Hawaiians, the image of a large islander is defined as an unhealthy body by its association with a medical discourse of pathology. I argue that other interpretations of large bodies also need to be considered.

Medicine and epidemiology are not the sole contributors to discourses of pathology and risk. As Turner (1996) has noted, medical efforts at constructing an "efficient body" are not just a matter of defining health as a goal of medicine, but also a moral and capitalist endeavor. This concept is furthered by Comaroff's 2007 argument that with neoliberalism the body becomes an individual representation of identity. As individual bodies are vested with identity they are "defined as objects of biological nature and subjects of commodified desire (p. 199)." In response we can imagine the incongruity of body size and its association with identity representations in Hawai'i. We are presented with the pathologically large Hawaiian body as defined by modern medical discourse, and the ubiquitous body image of tourism in the hula dancer. These two images represent the intersection of capitalism (i.e., a body defined as an object of biological nature) and morality (i.e., a body defined as a subject of commodified desire). Recalling the discussion of commodification, erasure of history, and hula in Chapter 3, the representation and interpretation of the hula dancer's body provides a striking parallel for examining how bodies are contested and reclaimed through colonizing discourses.[1] Hula's strong tie to the remembrance of Native Hawaiian ancestors and its use as a capitalist commodity in tourism constructs it as one of the most valued and contested bodies (e.g., Buck 1993; Trask 1993; Stillman 2001; Silva 2004).[2] Like the body of the hula dancer, representations of the Native Hawaiian body and its health are contested as both embodied memory and subject to control through moral and medical discourses. The centrality of the body as a "natural" object defined and disciplined by structural discourses, unevenly enacted in the United States, produce subjectivities for on- and off-islanders that reflect their desire to provide "healthier" representations of Hawaiian bodies with varying degrees of incorporation into the larger medicalized and capitalist discourse.

The fit or "healthy" body models are often used as evidence of physical capital (Bourdieu 1984) for both the individual and society at large. The large Hawaiian body, however, is out of control, undisciplined, and at risk. The poor practices and waste of the large Hawaiian body are marked as unproductive in a capitalist economy. For example, one evening a luna (supervisor or foreman) from a local pineapple field mentioned that the teenage son of his co-worker was so large that he was "unable to bend over to tie his shoe." "It must be hard," he said, "to be that unhealthy." He went on to describe how hard this boy found it to work in the fields and how he could barely complete a half-day's worth of labor. Unlike the images of Hawaiian bodies used for tourism that are productive as commodities, this young man's inability to be productive is directly linked to his health as symbolized by his large body size.

Drawing on Foucault, we could also interpret these representations and their embodiment as bodies disciplined through the technologies of power, whether it be through the demands of a tourist industry selling leisure and sex, or as risky, unhealthy bodies defined by the plethora of statistics, BMI values, fat intake, and the necessary amount of daily activity to be considered productive. Nevertheless, the exercise of power upon the body is still based within a U.S. middle-class understanding of self-control, production, and consumption (Crawford 1984). As Crawford argues, "health and the body imagined through it . . . are not only biological and practical but . . . paced with connotations about what it means to be good, respectable and responsible (1994:1348)." Health as a marker of identity is meaningful because of the creation of the "unhealthy" other (Crawford 1994; McMullin 2005). Thus, body projects that aim to cultivate a fit, healthy body can be interpreted as reflecting one's successful participation in the capitalist community. However, the "unhealthy" other, which is a large, fat body, can signify rejection of the need for physical capital and exclusion from capitalist projects. That this view is the primary interpretation of the body in general raises questions about discourses that contest the fit, healthy representation as the sole embodiment of capitalist production.

This chapter offers four interpretations of Hawaiian bodies: a productive and depoliticized body, an unproductive and pathologized body, a pathologized and politicized body, and finally the fit and politicized body. The last two bodies are alternative versions of representations that contest capitalist interpretations. The politicized bodies emphasize the agency of Native Hawaiians to rewrite the meanings associated with both the large Hawaiian body and the fit Hawaiian body. However, the point at which the healthy Hawaiian body is invested with the history of its ancestors, colonialism, inequality, and struggle and is re-vitalized with Hawaiian knowledge is precisely when the body is most susceptible to ideologies of diet, fitness, and capitalist consumption. In the case of the "Healthy Ancestor," there is a concern that the counter-hegemonic movement will be incorporated into the hegemonic discourses of medicine and physical fitness. They will become bodies that are desirable and lose the advantage of being a method of political critique. Likewise, discourses that promote health through physical fitness will continue to neglect a critique of the political economy that rewards the achievements of individually fit bodies.

The Productive and Depoliticized Body

Hawaiian sports figures like Olympic swimmer and surfer Duke Paoa Kahanamoku, or Lokelani McMichael, the eight-time Ironman triathlete, have often been a popular source of information about Native Hawaiians and the Hawaiian islands. Their success at achieving the pinnacle of fitness allows them to be represented as symbols of capitalist control, yet it also provides an avenue through which Native Hawaiian history and origins can be disseminated to the general population. For example, Duke Paoa Kahanamoku's success as an Olympic gold-medalist swimmer paved his entrée into global venues, which facilitated the sentiment that he was Hawai'i's ambassador and bearer

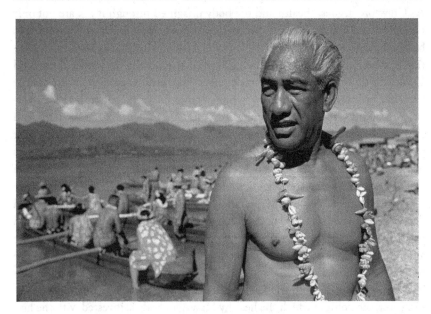

Figure 6.1. "Hawaiian Hero," 1955. Duke Paoa Kahanamoku (1890–1968) playing a Native Chief in the film "Mister Roberts." Kahanamoku was an Olympic swimming champion before his acting career and went on to serve as Honolulu's sheriff for 26 years. (Photo by Slim Aarons/Hulton Archive/Getty Images).

of knowledge of he'e nalu (surfing), thereby bringing it to broader audiences. The early history of he'e nalu, however, also reveals the practice as a protest against colonial efforts to control the male Hawaiian body (Walker 2008). The surf and surfing, according to Walker, is a space where Native Hawaiian men in particular, through clubs such as Hui Nalu and surfing competitions showed the colonists that ka po'ina nalu (the surf zone) was a domain controlled by Kanaka Maoli. Through their mastery of the ocean and their sport, surfers from the Hui Nalu, like Duke Kahanamoku, resisted efforts to characterize Hawaiian men as "submissive," but rather crafted their own representations as being "physically fit and strong, and several had reputations for being extremely tough" (Walker 2008:97). An emphasis on sports and the associated "physically fit" body are issues of control that are always embedded in power relations. What is debated is whether that control will be defined as located in individuals (an enlightenment view) or extended into the larger sphere of power relations (a political economy view).

The contemporary emphasis on fitness as a symbol of participation in the capitalist economy has facilitated the representation of the fit, athletic body as something to be consumed. Similar to the use of the hula dancer image to sell Hawai'i (see Chapter 2), the fit body is also used to sell products such as clothing, food, equipment, and videos that enhance the discipline and control of unruly bodies. One need only note the rapid increase of fitness and diet magazines, books, TV shows, and gyms over the past few decades to recognize the impact of this multibillion-dollar industry. Thus, the fit athletic body and its consumables slide easily into the meaning of health.

The link between exercise, health, and body size is evident in Pualani's response to my question asking her to describe a healthy person. Pualani is a 44-year-old homemaker who lives in California. While she does not have a regular fitness regimen she is by no means overweight. In her response she stated that:

> Hawaiians tend to be heavier. Our whole family is heavier. If they're not heavy they tend to stand out. Uhm, my mother's got nine brothers and sisters, and out of all nine of them there's one that isn't overweight. She's actually considered skinny. . . . So healthy Hawaiians usually are the younger ones. All my nieces and nephews they're swimming on the weekends, they're paddling on the weekends. My cousin is forty, probably about forty-four, and he canoes in a canoe club. He's very healthy. Because his stamina's really strong, his muscle tone is strong. He uhm, he's just active all the time. His weight is down. So he stands out too. And then I had a cousin that surfed. And while he was surfing he was in really good shape. But when he stopped, he's a little bit heavier. But I tend to think that the active ones don't tend to get as heavy. Because he was, I don't know if it was his image, because he

also has to keep his image up, because he has to do promotionals and stuff. He has to look good. He had a big name in surfing I guess.

Pualani begins her response by stating that "Hawaiians tend to be heavier." The pathology of the large body begins with the racial/ethnic categorization of Hawaiians. Anchoring the referent of fat to Hawaiians then permits her to move forward, comparing and contrasting the activity and productivity of her family. Throughout the rest of her description, weight is explicitly linked to health; a heavier body is a body at risk for disease. This risk, as Crawford (1984) would argue, can be mediated by controlling the body through fitness activities. Furthermore, this heavier risky body is not just linked to health, the physical form also embodies notions of Native Hawaiian identity, as evidenced by: "If they're not heavy, they tend to stand out." In this way the body is again used to differentiate Native Hawaiians from others. In categorizing Native Hawaiians and defining Hawaiian health, however, Pualani calls on the image of unruly heavy bodies as well as the fitness activities that can be used to control those bodies. What is particularly interesting is that she concludes with her cousin who, in her view, had maintained his health until he stopped surfing. Until that time, as a "big name in surfing" he was a productive body and the image of health. This image was a necessary component of his appeal as a body made for consumption. For Pualani, the link between health and body size for Native Hawaiians revolved around engagement in fitness activities. Through the contrasts of activity and fitness, large Hawaiian bodies are racialized as potentially healthy and yet failing, through their own lack of control, to achieve the bodily representation that signifies participation in an active life and the capitalist community.

The intersections of health, body, and fitness as larger symbols of participation in the capitalist economy can be further extended by examining the body image represented by Kiana Tom. During the 1990s Kiana Tom was a well-known fitness instructor; she had two fitness/body sculpting shows on ESPN ("BodyShaping") and on ESPN2 ("Kiana's Flex Appeal"). She has been on the cover of numerous sports, fitness, and popular magazines, and has a book on body sculpting. Kiana was born in Hawai'i, but was raised in southern California with the pedigree that is typical of Hawaiians: she is part Hawaiian, Chinese, and Irish. Kiana's name is Hawaiian for "calm water." Her body project is an image of health that is attained through the self-discipline of rigorous and consistent diet and exercise. What makes Kiana's body different from that of any other fitness guru is that she is framed by the exotic appeal of her island heritage. Her modern-day fitness and heritage are sold as a consumable for achieving health and sexuality that were also desired and controlled by early explorers, colonists, and contemporary tourists (Figure 6.1).

The implied naturalness of fit bodies, health, and consumption are made meaningful through their link to Hawai'i. This is achieved by calling our attention to her heritage as a Native Hawaiian and by locating the other half of the health dyad (exercise and diet) to the Hawaiian islands. She furthers her use of Hawaiian identity in her body-sculpting book by providing dietary advice and recipes. In the section titled "Kiana's Low-fat Hawaiian Cooking," she encourages us to try her diet plan by saying, "Try preparing these delicious Hawaiian specialties instead of the usual low-fat fare. This is the best way I know of to stay lean and still enjoy the sensual pleasure of eating. After all, eating is one of the pleasures in life." (Rosenthal and Tom 1994:132). Included in her "low fat Hawaiian recipes" are "Kona Banana egg whites, Island oatmeal, and Pineapple Chicken Maui Style." Ironically enough, the "Hawaiian" recipes do not recall the mana (life force) imbued in the land or the ancestors that occupy the land. Rather, her Hawaiianness and "Hawaiian" recipes draw on a remembrance of place; of islands, of Kona, of Maui as they are employed to sell pleasure, the exotic, a place that serves the needs of a conception of health that does not really need to be located. There is nothing particularly "Hawaiian" about egg whites or oatmeal, nor is there any allusion to the connection to Kona or Maui as places of the ancestors. Pineapple, however, recalls a history of colonization. It is a history of land grabbing by missionaries for their plantations, the diversion of water and other island resources, and the importation of laborers to work the fields, yet this is not the history that is sold. The food and the geographical place are connected because like the physical capital of Kiana's body, the places have become symbolic capital and symbols of leisure—"the sensual pleasure of eating" that awaits those who participate in healthy body projects.

Kiana is a self-disciplined, productive, and consumable body. While Kiana's diet and exercise plan may promote health represented by a trim body and nutritious diet, it is a secularized notion of health and diet that is not dependent on Hawaiian land. In other words, it is something that any individual can achieve if they only have the required self-discipline and control, regardless of the sociopolitical and colonial context. In doing so, the politics that created Hawai'i and Hawaiians as entities to be consumed are obscured through the body that is made fit with an eye toward longevity and sex appeal.

The Large Hawaiian Body and IZ: The Unproductive Pathologized and the Pathologized Politicized Body

Kiana's fit, productive Hawaiian body is a startling contrast to the image of the large Hawaiian body. The 700-pound body of the late and popular Native Hawaiian singer Israel Kamakawiwo'ole, or IZ as he was more commonly known, was used by Keoni to illustrate the embodiment of Hawaiian attitudes.[3] Keoni is a 45-year-old male who was raised in Hawai'i but left the islands to attend college in California. Currently, he is very active in promoting Hawaiian cultural events in California. During our conversation he was very enthusiastic about reviving and teaching Hawaiians "traditional" and contemporary farming techniques so they could support themselves. This enthusiasm, however, was directed at Hawaiians living "at home." Again, we see the role of geographic place in terms of identifying *which* bodies need to learn specific practices. In addition, he was very critical of present cultural attitudes of Hawaiian health. According to Keoni, Hawaiians adored IZ because his body and songs represented the hopelessness of the Hawaiian situation. As he told me, IZ was a Hawaiian body out of control; he was obese, had no control over his food intake, he sang about the plight of Hawaiians, making them feel like they also have no control over their land or their situation. IZ shows Hawaiians that they cannot control the situation they are in exactly because of that attitude. Thus, in Keoni's opinion, Hawaiians identify with IZ. He went on to say that because Hawaiians feel like they have no control so they do not do anything about their health. According to this representation IZ becomes the pathological body for Keoni.

As we take a second look at IZ, his body and actions suggest a different interpretation, that of a politicized body, albeit a body that is simultaneously pathologized. One of the songs Keoni used to exemplify IZ's lyrics regarding the plight of Hawaiians was *Hawai'i 78* (1993). This song was frequently played on the radio when I was conducting fieldwork in Hawai'i. The song begins with the call "Ua mau, ke ea o ka 'Āina, I ka pono, 'o Hawai'i" (The sovereignty of the land has been continued because it is pono ~ translation Silva 2004). IZ continues to sing about how the early monarchs would feel if they saw the islands now, with the desecration of sacred grounds and the massive development of present-day cities in Hawai'i. This vision of the cities described in *Hawai'i 78*, he indicates, would be a source of great pain for the monarchy, the land, and the people. Although Keoni viewed this song as the embodiment of the hopelessness of the Hawaiian people, many consider it to be an anthem of the sovereignty movement. Interestingly, the official lyrics to this song, elaborated on in the version that was played on the radio and is on the CD, *Facing Future* (1993), tell a more personal story of his family, his father's struggles, his own struggles, and how his father came back to him as a spirit to tell him to let people help him with his drug and depression problems. This form of "talking story" interjected with the theme of *Hawai'i 78* conveys a feeling of crisis in the Hawaiian nation (What would our ancestors think if they saw what has happened), as well as a sense of crisis in the individual life of this particular Native Hawaiian. That the spirit of IZ's father came back to advise and guide IZ again links the daily lives of Hawaiians to the ancestors in the ways we care for land and body. It is also important to note his use of "Ua mau, ke ea o ka 'Āina, I ka pono, 'o Hawai'i," words first spoken by Kamehameha IV and translated by Silva (2004:37) as "The sovereignty of the land has been continued because it is pono."IZ's use of Kamehameha IV's words is not simply a reference to the state motto; it can be interpreted as a recognition of where Native Hawaiian sovereignty lies. The crisis in this song and in his life offers an opportunity for many to identify with him in the pain of loss of land and sovereignty in Hawai'i, while he simultaneously calls for a return to a "proper"way of life, to pono.

As IZ's and Kiana's bodies are used to represent opposite extremes of the ideals of health, they both integrate conceptions of Hawaiian land into their body projects. The juxtaposition of the meaning of land for IZ and Kiana reveal that for the fit, sculpted body Hawaiian land is disembodied; it is a place that is used to sell a vision of health that can easily travel the globe (McMullin 2005). However, for IZ land is embodied with the strength, struggles, memories, and more importantly, the mana of the ancestors. The land, through its genealogical link to Native Hawaiians, is personified (e.g., Kame'eleihiwa 1992; Silva 2004).

I mentioned Keoni's interpretation of IZ as a Hawaiian body out of control to a friend living in Hawai'i and she was saddened by his response and completely disagreed with it, saying that IZ represented hope; his songs were about the joy and pride of being Hawaiian. They address our current struggles and point us forward. She went on to state that "he reminds us of our ancestors." In that, she found great solace and knew that she must continue the struggle. This sentiment was also expressed by Native Hawaiians quoted in Marshall's 2006 work on revitalizing Hawaiian pride. One of her participant's reveals the profound impact of this song on how she imagined Hawaiian history, stating that his music moved her to "think beyond Western myths of Hawai'i, to remember a different past and conjure a different present" (Marshall 2006:194).

The interpretation of IZ as a source of hope is also alluded to on the cover of the album *Facing Future* in which we see IZ with his back turned toward us. The future he is facing is not the one that capitalist control has offered; rather, as the historian Kame'eleihiwa states:

It is as if the Hawaiian stands firmly in the present, with his back to the future, and his eyes fixed upon the past, seeking historical answers for present-day dilemmas. Such an orientation is to the Hawaiian an eminently practical one, for the future is always unknown, whereas the past is rich in glory and knowledge (1992:22).

These contrasting views highlight the complexities involved in giving meaning to the body; between recognition of the sociopolitical contexts that frame

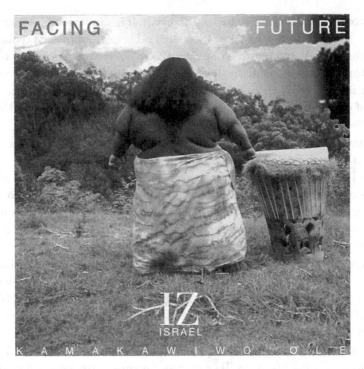

Figure 6.2.   Album: *Facing Future*, Artist: Israel IZ Kamakawiwoʻole. Courtesy of Mountain Apple Company Hawaii, www.mountainapplecompany.com

the health of Native Hawaiians and the conflation of the body as individual control over health. IZ's struggles with his weight and drug problems, his enduring love and happiness for the people and family, and his support for sovereignty made him a beloved symbol for Native Hawaiians in Hawaiʻi and in California. But also, especially for Keoni, IZ was a symbol of an unhealthy body, a body out of control. For some people, IZ's presumed lack of a body project and the image of his obese body overshadowed what he had to say in his music, leading to a different interpretation of his lyrics. Despite the fact that his music was productive and made money, despite his calls to sovereignty, to pono, and to remember the ancestors, IZ's body size was used in a clearly contradictory way by Keoni. Keoni used IZ to suggest a pathological body, a hopeless body; one that was not a participant in capitalist consumption and therefore not productive.[4]

IZ's body serves as a point of disagreement. Is his a body out of control, as Keoni would have us believe? Or, as Scheper-Hughes and Lock (1987) might argue, is he a representation of the *mindful body*, one that has recognized inequalities inherent in capitalism, and has resisted, refusing to participate in a system that is designed to devalue his people? Through its size, the large Hawaiian body calls our attention to resistance against the economic and social inequities evident in the lives of Native Hawaiians. If the controlled, fit, healthy body is a sign of all that is good about capitalism, is the unhealthy, large body a sign of all that is bad? It is not enough to place large bodies outside of capitalism because they are a product of consumption, albeit of over-consumption. It is also not enough to call attention to the fact that it is a risky body, with Native Hawaiians having some of the highest rates of obesity in the nation, a body that is potentially pathological because of its ability to contract the wide array of diseases that science has suggested and society has deemed as inevitable. Given the remembrance of the ancestors evident in IZ's songs I would suggest that his body is a *mindful body* or, more appropriately, he is a "revolting body" (LeBesco 2004). Calling our attention to the political nature of fat, LeBesco (2004) uses the term "revolting bodies" to discuss the projects through which fat activists resignify the spoiled identities attached to fat. In the same vein, I am arguing for a resignification of large Native Hawaiian bodies, that is, a transition from a racialized failed body to that of a resistant, *revolting body*. Rather than a body out of control, large Hawaiian bodies signify inequality and are in revolt against the historical, political, and economic inequities experienced by Native Hawaiians. Moreover, the *revolting body* remembers ancestors, a past and future that is situated in the land and restores one to pono, to health. Viewing large bodies as an embodied revolt against the political and economic inequities faced by Native Hawaiians also suggests agency by asking us to reconsider the assumed egalitarian and naturalness of healthy and unhealthy identities. In the largeness of his body, IZ can speak to us about the land and history of Hawai'i. Yet, our capitalist discourse makes it easier to view IZ's body as a body out of control rather than as a body in revolt. As a result his message is complicated by American ideologies of individualism, control, and the medicalization of the body, contesting his voice and obscuring it through the naturalization of power on the body. The body image of IZ demands that we rethink the meaning of large bodies. Most people, Hawaiian or not, who know of IZ reflect first on his music; his voice is first and foremost in our hearts and minds. For people not raised in Hawai'i or in the Pacific, for that matter, the size of his body often consumes our attention. There is a presumed disconnect between the beauty of his songs and the pathology of his body. It is precisely this disconnect, however, that forces us to re-evaluate him; it allows us to move away from a meaning of pathology into a meaning of resistance and revolt. Thus, the expansive body and the music that calls Hawaiians to remember their ancestors both invite us to consider the exercise of power in the Islands—the sources of inequality and the knowledge necessary to reconfigure a political economy that characterizes Native Hawaiians as "naturally" unhealthy.

The Fit Hawaiian Body: Productive and Politicized

Although the resistant, "revolting" fat body has significant forces contesting its meaning, the image of the Healthy Ancestor is another symbol that disputes both the meaning of health and the stereotypes of Native Hawaiians as being unhealthy. The contested nature of Hawaiian land and cultural knowledge is reflected in the larger historical and social discourse on Native Hawaiian health (Blaisdell 1989; McMullin 2005). Also, against the socio-historical context of the depopulation, Māhele, and subsequent overthrow of the Hawaiian monarchy, once again, the image of the Healthy Ancestor is a symbol that disputes both the meaning of health and stereotypes of Native Hawaiians as unhealthy (McMullin 2005). The Healthy Ancestor motivates and inspires Native Hawaiians to integrate their health and culture, to pono and lōkahi. For many of the Native Hawaiians I spoke with, looking back to the lifestyles of their ancestors is one of the key aspects to becoming healthy again, and ultimately to focus on and resolve the economic contradictions in their lives.

The fit Native Hawaiian body, like productive bodies, is also linked to food and land in specific ways. However, the foods that are manifested in the body are historicized, focused on transformation, linked to the land and, as discussed in the previous chapters, healthy Hawaiians are a product of the land. Additives and processed foods have transformed the Hawaiian body as it becomes more like the bodies of foreigners: alienated from the land and, as a result, no longer healthy. Whereas Kiana Tom's Hawaiian diet used representations of geographic place for control and consumption, Lani's vision of a healthy diet takes geographic place as a location of an ongoing struggle between the introduction of foreign values and the practices of living off the land:

> Hawaiians healthy? Like before? No there's not much because of the . . . our ways of life is so changed. It's not like before, where we could go in the taro patch and do, you know. Before it used to be fun going in the patches and working, but the kids are so modernized now that they look at you like "what for?" You know, "I can pick up everything I need in the store. I don't have to go to the mountains or to the oceans or whatever." There are very few that you'll find that will do that. . . . 'Cause when they were younger we could, you know, go all over the place and enjoy. Now you can't because either crosses somebody's property, or you can't go here, or you cannot go down the beach anymore. You know, can't go without having permits or things like that. So, we, we're losing a whole lot. And our children are, and now

by the time they're have their own family it won't be the same unless we can get it back. Other than that we lose everything. We, we the one that losing everything. No more the healthy life anymore.

Historicizing and linking health and food back to the land destabilizes representations that seek to naturalize the contemporary health of Native Hawaiians as a stable category outside any social and political context. In an effort to attend to these contradictions, the use of the Healthy Ancestor as a symbol of health reconfigures a body project that fully incorporates and acknowledges historical and political meanings associated with geographical place and identity. The image of the Healthy Ancestor not only links Native Hawaiians to land and food but is bolstered by a body image that reflects ideals of fitness and health. The authors of *The Wai'anae Book of Hawaiian Health* (Shintani and Hughes 1993), dispute representations that naturalize the poor health and obesity of contemporary Native Hawaiians by referencing observations of early explorers that paint a picture of the beauty of ancient Hawaiians. Using the observations of one early observer made in 1832, they state that:

> The Hawaiian people were tall, "above the middle stature, . . . graceful and . . . stately." They were attractive and healthy. This was the conclusion of an early observer in times soon after Western contact. Hawaiian people today have it in them to be this way, if we return to some of the ways of our *kupuna*. (Shintani and Hughes 1993:9)

The *Book of Hawaiian Health* promotes the idea that Native Hawaiians can achieve the health and beauty of their ancestors by returning to the diet of their ancestors. The image of a Hawaiian nation is that of healthy, graceful people living off the land, eating a diet that was passed down to them through the generations, and a diet that they must now struggle to regain. Reports by the early explorers are combined with photos to reinforce the observations that in the past Native Hawaiians "were thin and not overweight" (Shintani and Hughes 1993). Even though these images are presented through the reports of early explorers and colonists, and as such, attend to the bodily form with foreign values, they are used here to contest contemporary views that naturalize the size and assumed poor health of Native Hawaiians.

The body of the healthy Hawaiian ancestor is used as an image to motivate and inspire Hawaiians to integrate their health and culture, to pono; to reconnect the fit body with food and land. As Shintani and Hughes note in the section on Kino:

> Kino (body) represents the physical side of life. We are connected to our food. This is one way in which the principle of "ola lōkahi" (oneness with life) pertains to our

bodies. It was a basic understanding of ancient Hawaiians that food, land, water, and health were inseparable. It was believed that all foods had a life force, and that eating food was sustaining health by adding the life force to the body. (1993:34)

Food unlike Kiana's diet plan is more than a location that evokes sensuality; in this case, it evokes a life force, a belonging to the land that cannot be displaced without adverse consequences to health. More importantly, as these researchers note in the principles of eating, one must, "express your gratitude before eating and understand that you are connected to the ʻāina through the mana of your food" (Shintani and Hughes 1993:42). The integration of identity in this diet program, unlike Kiana's diet program, is firmly rooted in the socio-historical context of Native Hawaiians' experience and knowledge, and not capitalist consumption.

This is not to say that the vision of the Healthy Ancestor is not complicated by the realities of what many people see around them. While Islanders recognize that obesity is a problem for many of their peers, that recognition is contrasted with the healthy bodies of the generations before. As Mokihana, a woman who prides herself on being 100 percent Native Hawaiian noted:

But it's the things that I've heard. . . . The foreigners that came into this country they happened to get that disease action. So, Hawaiians like they never had to take immunizations or anything . . . after everything was done [the introduction of diseases] I think that they stayed healthy, you know, strong enough. I mean the men before were built they were awesome looking you know. The men were solid people. The women were big. And you look at them now, ho, it's just the opposite [laughs], and all the wahines [women] all come skinny and the men are braless [laughs]. So it's quite a change.

Like Keoni she recognizes size as a problem, but the large body is now rooted in a history of colonization and disease. The body, whether beautiful and stately, or a man who is so fat he requires a bra symbolizes the profoundly negative social transformations that have occurred in the Hawaiian islands. Furthermore, her observations reflect the gendered effects of colonization on bodies.[5] Women's bodies are thin, controlled, and disciplined for an ideal sexualized selling of island life (Buck 1993; Trask 1993; Desmond 1999). Like Kiana's body, the kind of feminine body that society wants and needs is thin, sexually appealing, beautiful—revealing itself as the embodiment of capitalist desires of control and self-discipline. The thin feminized body combined with colonial and neo-colonial desires to control the exotic islander create an ideal for women's bodies that is not as clear for men's bodies. The braless men, in contrast, are left unattended, with no specific task in the capitalist community. In a capitalist interpretation of body control, men's bodies, like IZ's body, are neither desired nor valued as absolutely necessary for labor. Indeed, as Walker (2008) argues, it was the desire of the Whites on island to characterize Hawaiian men as ineffectual.

Mokihana's description of this gendered shift in body size reflects yet another racialized contradiction resulting from the capitalist encounter. The obese body is not simply unproductive and out of control, it is a body that is transformed from what once was strong and healthy. In this case the obese body is the negative *result* of the forces of capitalism and colonialism, which have denied individuals the ability to define the meaning and practices that constitute productive bodies. By focusing on the historical contrast, Mokihana acknowledges the medical discourse on obesity while denaturalizing the current representations of Hawaiian health.

Complicating the Fit Hawaiian Body

In the end we have a fit image of health for both capitalist consumption and control, and Native Hawaiian resistance and revival. One body is achieved through self-discipline and is the embodiment of capitalist production and consumption; the other is achieved through the practices of pre-contact ancestors and is the embodiment of social relationships past and present. Interestingly, in the late 1990s Dateline NBC produced a segment on the "Hawaiian diet." With the 100-year observance of the overthrow of the monarchy in 1893, and annexation in 1898, there had been a significant rise in efforts by the Native Hawaiian sovereignty movements to call attention to the history and politics of these events. The efforts to educate the American public on the illegal overthrow of a sovereign kingdom also gave rise to a renewed interest in all things Hawaiian, particularly on the mainland. The segment on the Hawaiian diet on Dateline NBC was yet another contribution to a discourse that sought to define the Hawaiian identity. The program touted the success of returning to a diet of fish, poi, and limu. It showed pictures of the fit "thin" body of ancient Hawaiians and the large obese bodies of contemporary Hawaiians. The interviews included a Native Hawaiian woman who had participated in the diet, as well as an interview with Dr. Shintani. The success of the diet was acknowledged through research that showed increased weight loss, reduced cholesterol levels, and control of diabetes (so much so that individuals were able to discontinue the use of insulin) (Shintani et al. 1991). Furthermore, the Dateline program concluded by showing how one can adapt the diet to any locale, again demonstrating that health practices are transportable; for example, one could replace kalo with broccoli. What is particularly useful is that in this extension, the diet could be both culturally meaningful and practical for off-islanders. It clearly provides alternatives for individuals who cannot access foods such as kalo, pōhole, and limu either because of lack of availability or financial cost. It is a positive effort at crafting opportunities for all Hawaiians to be healthy and to perpetuate Hawaiian values. But herein lies the rub: those aspects of the diet that made it distinctly Hawaiian, the ways in which Native Hawaiians are tied to the land through food, water, and genealogy that Shintani clearly supports, are not mentioned in the NBC program as yet another diet product becomes available for larger global consumption. Although the segment was taped in Hawai'i, and images of the Healthy Ancestor were promoted, the importance of health through a tangible connection to the embodied land was not viewed as part of what the American public needed to know. All the scientific information needed to live a healthy life was presented to the viewers. The "Hawaiian diet" may have made it to prime time, but the political message was lost in the way in which it was secularized and marketed for the general population.

In a Focauldian sense, the body is normalized, disciplined through medicalization into secular morals of fitness and diet. It is from this transformation that Turner's 1992 argument stems, that is, of the "growth of a consumer society with its emphasis on the athletic/beautiful body"—a diet for the management of the spirit and soul as a Hawaiian diet would prescribe, is transformed into diet for the purposes of longevity and sexuality as is seen through medicalization in mortality statistics and the fit controlled body of Kiana. Thus, to the extent that it can be claimed that the healthy Hawaiian body is the product of individual self-discipline and not linked to the social, economic, and political alienation of Hawaiians from their land, efforts to use the Healthy Hawaiian to promote Native Hawaiian identity and sovereignty will continue to be obscured. The alternative meaning of being a sovereign healthy Hawaiian is susceptible to control by a capitalist, self-disciplined body.

An examination of the body and its use as a signifier of health clarifies the work of power relationships on yet another *natural* category. Similar to the processes of globalization, biomedical views of health require a decontextualized perception of the body. In other words, bodies can perform labor, culture, gender, and health in any location. Examining the meaning of the corporeal body, which is at the center of "health," allows for additional examination of the process of power through the political economy and identity formation. Unlike identities that are fluid and positioned, the physical body is taken to be the same physical entity regardless of the context and location in which it is positioned. For enlightenment views and current neoliberal practices to work effectively, it must be assumed that physical bodies remain the same in the process of migration, moving from context to context. Because body and health are believed to be mobile, the same rules apply to all bodies and all efforts to achieve health. The fit athletic body and the unfit obese body, the corporeal form and the foods that constitute them, reference a geographical place that in a capitalist reading can be used to sell. Kiana and IZ are racialized bodies that reference Hawai'i and Hawaiian food and culture. These references, while part of what make the body alluring and/or disgusting, are simply background to global bodies and goods that would appear in and out of control despite their locale. The body itself is still a biological form, malleable to biomedical interventions, and desirous of health. As a consequence, both capitalist consumption and biomedical hegemony are nurtured by the process of naturalizing and globalizing the body and health.

These global expectations and complexities of body are contested by Native Hawaiians' definition of health. The connection between land, food, body, and health is fused in such a manner that it is difficult to talk about one without the other and all reference different facets of Hawaiianness. Whether we examine a revolting body or the fit body of the ancestors, Native Hawaiians reference the land and historical struggles, and provide a clear sign of what it means to be Native Hawaiian. Hawaiian land as a referent for health rejects the global notion that health can be decontextualized. The body of the ancestors also rejects notions that Native Hawaiians are "naturally" unhealthy. In focusing on these supposed natural categories, however, we must also ascertain that health and body are not subsumed through a medicalizing discourse that also seeks to return Native Hawaiians to health, but without their land or a recognition of how politics frames the contemporary milieu.

Endnotes

1. Important research on the political, historical, and contemporary meaning of hula has been conducted by scholars such as Kaeppler (1993), Stillman (1998, 2002), and Silva (2004).
2. Buck's (1993) and Silva's (2004) excellent work show how throughout the history of Kanaka struggles, hula is used to tell the history stories of Kanaka origins and genealogy. As such, hula is a symbol of resistance to colonial and neocolonial hegemony.
3. IZ died in 1997. Prior to his death it was said that he was 6 feet 2 inches tall and weighed approximately 757 pounds.
4. After IZ's death his rendition of "Somewhere Over the Rainbow"/"What a Wonderful World" was used in an etoys commercial and during an episode of the TV drama ER, as well as in other settings. More recently (2006), in an ironic twist for health, IZ's music was used in a commercial for Rice Krispies.
5. See also Green (2002) for an excellent discussion of the colonization of Native Hawaiian female bodies.

CONCLUSION: INEQUALITY, HEALTH, AND IDENTITY

Contributions to a Critical Medical Anthropology Approach

Critical medical anthropology (CMA) has long recognized that biomedical and enlightenment views fall short of crafting "healthy" bodies. Baer, Singer, and Susser (2003:5) have noted that "health is not some absolute state of being but an elastic concept that must be evaluated in a larger socio-cultural context." Part of that larger context includes the role of cultural identity in supporting or challenging medical hegemonies. Examining the intersections between health and cultural identity helps to denaturalize biomedical definitions of health and moves us toward including knowledge that is based on a shared history of sovereignty, capitalist encounters, resistance, and integrated innovation.

Thus, a political economy of health approach frames the interpretation and debate over health and how to achieve it. This work has elaborated on facets of power relations that are naturalized and de-naturalized through health discourses and identity politics. These contributions include historical and current Hawaiian knowledge of health; which enables us to see the cultural aspects of biomedical hegemony and the structural processes at work making it appear as if it has no cultural basis. When we fail to acknowledge how biomedicine is culture-based, then differences in health status or health inequalities are discussed as if they are a cultural problem or individual failing. More importantly, this work shows how Hawaiian knowledge forms the basis of a different set of techniques, practices, and relationships for health and in doing so it is also a critique of health inequalities and the capitalist ideologies that support inequity. The entry into Native Hawaiian knowledge of health reveals the elasticity of the health concept as a critique of capitalism and as a charter for good health among on- and off-islanders.

CMA also seeks to incorporate social and individual experience into our understanding of medicine. The critique of medical hegemony, in the case of Hawai'i, stems from the lived experience of Native Hawaiians and the greater burden of disease that they carry. Native Hawaiians' experience of health inequalities provide as well as push the imperative to call attention to the ways in which Western discourses naturalize health, body, and land such that the unequal distribution of resources and the ideologies that dismiss and denigrate other knowledges are made evident and opened to critique. This is not to say that the Native Hawaiian definition of health does not draw on a biosocial aspect that looks to their origin as a source of health; rather, by pointing out the fluidity of health as a symbol for cultural identity we see the contingency and positioning of the communities engaging in the power struggle to define health and to have access to resources that encourage a state of health.

The relationship between Native Hawaiian health and cultural identity pose intriguing questions about the naturalness of health, body, food, and land, and the politics of health inequities that are prevalent among most minority populations. Much of the work in the political economy of health and structural violence (for example, see Farmer 1999, 2003; Nguyen and Peschard 2003; Briggs and Mantini-Briggs 2003; Singer 2008; Baer 2008) has highlighted the relationships between globalization, neoliberal policies, and poor health. My work here contributes to this literature by focusing on the interrelationships between the meanings of place, health, and cultural identity as they are foregrounded in the health inequalities experienced by Native Hawaiians living on- and off-island. If we examine the physical attributes of health and body, then we can recognize how biomedical views of individual health and healing are linked to and informed by the processes of globalization, including migration and the construction of transnational identities. A Foucauldian view suggests that the current medical hegemony focuses on the "normality" of the body, proper technology, and medications, so that health and healing can take place in nearly any context. Combined with Enlightenment goals of alleviating human suffering through normalization disciplinary techniques are implemented through the medicalizing and homogenizing effects of colonial and current neoliberal policies (Heurtin-Roberts 2008). This decontextualized view of health separates people, and in this case Native Hawaiians, from geographical place and the identities that arise out of links with knowledge of their origins, both of place and ancestry. Extending this idea into the processes of globalization, scholars have noted that there is an emphasis on deterritorializing nations, people, and culture (Gupta and Ferguson 1992). As a result we have, on the one hand, a naturalizing process that through globalization and biomedicine can locate body, health, and food as timeless categories that have and will exist in different geographic locations. On the other hand, and more importantly, the naturalness that decontextualizes the body also obscures the sources of health inequalities, which can range from toxic environments and structural barriers to inadequate nutrition and medical technologies. A decontextualized view makes poor health a product of individual choices and practices, a lack of knowledge, or possession of erroneous "folk" knowledge, rather than a result of social inequalities de-linked from places of health.

Addressing health inequalities requires political rallying on the part of the disenfranchised and those who are in solidarity with them. The rallying cry for improving the health of Native Hawaiians contests discourses that naturalize poor health and pathologizes their bodies. More importantly, their own concern over health includes a clear action, through cultural, economic, and political sovereignty, that redresses the subjugation of their knowledge, and how these particular processes define who they are as a population (as discussed in Chapters 2 and 4). Through this process of redefinition, the remembering of the ancestors and the struggles over knowledge, land, food, and family, another kind of naturalizing process emerges. It is a naturalness that traces its existence through the generations and fuses Native Hawaiian identity with the land—it is a position that seeks to revitalize cultural *minds* that are securely linked to revitalized cultural *bodies*. Native Hawaiians, on- and off-island, find themselves positioned between the naturalness of these opposing ideals. The preceding chapters have described this positioning of identity through the examination of health, and the contested knowledge of land and body as they become symbols of health.

Another aspect of discourses that pathologize Native Hawaiian bodies focuses on the rapid and devastating loss of Native Hawaiian lives following the arrival of Europeans and Americans. The colonial view of these events is that Native bodies were unable to survive the rapid transformations brought to the islands. The history of Native Hawaiian health, however, reveals a continual struggle that reframes the political economy for biomedical as well as Native Hawaiian meanings of health. Furthermore, this meaning and the associated discourses of health proceed into the present, documenting and intervening in the health problems that plague the Native population. The recognition that Native Hawaiians have higher rates of chronic diseases than any other population in the state sets the stage for the counter-hegemonic discourse, which presents an altogether different narrative and understanding of Hawaiian health. Drawing on the same events that document the tragic loss of life, this opposing narrative does not view Native Hawaiians as a "naturally" unhealthy people. In fact, through the examination of their historical context (accounts of early explorers and studies of Hawaiian paleopathology; Trembly 1997) and looking back to the livelihoods of their ancestors we see that

Native Hawaiians were relatively healthy. By our standards of health—a good diet, regular exercise, and a fit body—Kanaka Maoli had achieved what we continually strive for today. This achievement was accomplished through recognizing social relationships with people, food, and land rather than the individual responsibility, knowledge of how to acquire proper health documents, and wealth that our current system promotes. Prior to colonial encounters, the ancestors had not experienced a massive depopulation as the result of infectious diseases, nor were they experiencing the chronic diseases that disproportionately affect them today. This alternative Hawaiian discourse highlights the colonial social and political practices that created the conditions in which poor health could flourish. The introduction of capitalist modes of production resulted in the subsequent alienation of the Native Hawaiians from the land and their methods of subsistence, and the subjugation of their knowledge. Many argue that these social transformations are what cause agents of disease and syndemics to take hold, and not a "naturally" weak body. The documentation and comparison of contexts, between pre- and post-contact, provide the knowledge to make efforts to improve health and reinforce a positive cultural identity. The Native Hawaiian cultural memory provides the details, from the Kumulipo (Hawaiian origin story) to the Wai'anae Comprehensive Health Program, that are believed to be keys in returning Native Hawaiians to a strong and healthy status. The counter-hegemonic discourse of what it means to be a healthy Hawaiian is defined by the people and is important for cultural identity and transforming present-day inequities.

Health-seeking practices are similarly caught up in a dual discourse of health and body as a natural symbol. The dominant discourse of public health and biomedicine questions why Native Hawaiians do not comply with the recommendations for health. The health "problem" is again framed in terms of individual failings rather than the economic and structural obstacles encountered in obtaining health care. Even more than the structural barriers, there is, at times, a preference for Hawaiian medical treatments. Not using the technologies of biomedicine is not always an example of non-compliance; in fact, I found that on-islanders used a combination of healing practices and were engaged in active resistance to biomedicine and a redefinition of the value of Native Hawaiian medical practices. Their resistance to biomedicine was not always a comment on the perceived efficacy of the treatments. Rather, resistance was against the complete integration of practices (i.e., amount of time doctors spent talking with patients and the plethora of insurance forms) into the market economy. They may reject the premises of biomedicine but still use it because of its efficacy, convenience (easy access to practitioners and medicinals), despite the constraints of insurance companies. Because of the demands of insurance companies, documents required in the practice of biomedicine and even the control of the body in the medical offices (i.e., signing in, waiting to be taken to the exam room, amount of time given to each patient), we can argue that a Foucauldian form of resistance to the technologies of power is taking place. Resistance, however, is not the only power relationship in play.

Hawaiian medical treatments are often used in conjunction with biomedicine, even while the Hawaiian treatments were viewed as a "purer" way of restoring health. Ideologically, biomedicine is treated as a proxy for Western ways and thus health-seeking behaviors reveal the struggle to revive Native Hawaiian ways against the current hegemony. Economically and practically, however, biomedicine is a convenient method for achieving physical health, but not necessarily cultural health or lōkahi. Revitalizing health through behaviors reveals the practical struggles between "Hawaiian ways," access to care, and the desire to feel well. The dynamics of resisting perceptions of non-compliance and redefining Native Hawaiian medical practices highlight the fluidity of identity for on- and off-islanders. The on-islanders' position was primarily but not solely opposed to biomedical treatments. Rather, they recognized areas of efficacy in both schools of medicine, rejecting the pathologizing, negative discourse of biomedicine and putting into practice Native Hawaiian ways of obtaining care. Thus, although different from the demands of biomedicine, their actions were not only resistance but an innovative integration of Hawaiian forms of health that can potentially negate or ignore biomedicine.

In contrast, off-islanders' experiences of health care in relation to Native Hawaiian medicine were constrained by their context; with no practitioners of Hawaiian medicine easily available, there was no position to take in relation to biomedicine. They simply did not have the options for healing that their on-islander counterparts did. The fluidity of Hawaiianness in these cases also reveals the workings of power in conjunction with the hegemonic discourses and structural support (insurance, biomedical technologies, access). Even if there was a counter-hegemonic discourse involving the use of Hawaiian medical practitioners off-island, there were no mechanisms in place to reconfigure the power relations associated with biomedicine.

Remembering Ancestors

The motivational force of remembering historical events and ancestors coupled with economic and geographical constraints influenced the relative salience of health as a symbol of cultural identity for on- and off-islanders. The symbol of the Healthy Ancestor is significant as an ideal for Native Hawaiian health because studies have shown that a return to the diet of the Hawaiian ancestors has a positive influence on the health of contemporary Hawaiians. This diet ideally entails having access to the 'āina, to Hawaiian land. Reviving the centrality of land in the lives of ancient and contemporary Native Hawaiians simultaneously forces us to remember their colonial encounters and their status as a "strong and healthy people." The history that is imbued in the Healthy Ancestor metaphor forces issues of sovereignty to the forefront. To talk about the Healthy Ancestor is to also talk about the ways in which Hawaiians became unhealthy and how they can become healthy again. The symbol of the Healthy Ancestor, while extremely important for defining health, is not viewed in the same way by on- and off-islanders. Because they could see their genealogy in the food and land right in front of them, on-islanders were reminded daily of the link between health and who they are as a people. In contrast, off-islanders who are removed from these daily reminders use other symbols to remember their ancestors: learning hula, language, maintaining contacts with their families on-island, and creating Native Hawaiian communities on the mainland. For off-islanders definitions of health were not so easily linked to the land and their ancestors. Instead they remembered the poor health of Hawaiians when they left the islands. Their own health practices included eating a healthy diet of fruits and vegetables, exercise, and maintaining positive relationships. Geographic boundaries made it difficult to find items such as kalo or pōhole, food from Hawaiian land. The symbols that are relevant for a Native Hawaiian conceptualization of health were not easily imported to the mainland. Their transnational identities involved more than just recreating the ideals of the homeland, they reflected their position in relation to the dominant health discourses that were available to them. Off-islander subjectivities were not tied to the land in the same way; however, they did engage in those aspects of Hawaiian identity that allowed them to remember their ancestors through bodies that enacted Hawaiian values. In this way they become the living 'āina, caring for themselves is caring for the ancestors.

Representations of health often found their most poignant form in the body. Through on-islanders' discourses of health they remembered the ancestors and their historical and contemporary economic and political struggles. Indeed, even through the corpulence corpulent of their bodies, they screamed revolt against the economic contradictions that capitalist encounters had imposed upon them. The prevalent capitalist ideals of body see normalcy as fit, controlled, and productive. The pathological body is viewed as obese, uncontrolled, and unproductive. In contrast, Native Hawaiian ideals see a healthy body as fit, but that body must also be intimately tied with the land and the ancestors. In the process of naturalizing bodies, the ideals of land can become subsumed in our desire to consume. In an effort to appeal to a contemporary emphasis on consuming health products as a symbol of participation in a capitalist community, a link to land was invoked. However, in the tourist and consumption discourse, Hawai'i as a sensual place of leisure where one can achieve health was devoid of the meaning attached to land by Native Hawaiians. The way in which Native Hawaiians link land, health, body, and identity depends on recognizing the genealogical ties one has to the ancestors and to the land. Herein we also see a dual naturalizing process applied to the body. Enlightenment views as well as capitalism and neoliberalism claims to the body demand that its normal state is to be healthy, of normal size (as defined currently by BMI), and free of disease, and more importantly that the body, like health, does not need to be contextualized. What is healthy for one is healthy for all, no matter the time and place. In direct opposition to those premises, Native Hawaiians' claim that Native bodies are healthy when they are free to live on the land of their ancestors; to mālama 'āina and the land will care for you. Defining health for Native Hawaiians is to recognize the context, the struggle, the place, and the time when their ancestors were healthy.

Recognizing the hegemonic power being exercised through current discourses of health does not imply that Native Hawaiian discourses of health are devoid of the exercise of power. Following Foucault, I argue that all relationships are infused with power and resistance. But is the recognition of the naturalizing process and the exercise of power in these competing knowledges the only point we can make? Recall Das's 1990 quote that appeared in the introduction:

> We have to see how we may define health so that instead of becoming a measure of the normal and the pathological, a means by which power may be exercised upon the one who declares that he is in pain, it becomes a means for the practices of freedom (1990:43).

If we read the ongoing health and sovereignty debate only as a reaction to biomedicine and capitalism then we have resistance. And yet, it is clear that there is so much more going on in the emphasis on a different set of social relationships. Native Hawaiians are working towards disentangling themselves from the current status quo; by reminding us of historical and current encounters that have resulted in a plethora of health problems, Native Hawaiians have declared that they are in pain. In defining health on their own terms and telling us how to restore health, Native Hawaiians are calling for the "means for the practices of freedom" separate from the current practices of health. Recognizing the contexts in which social inequalities produce health inequalities is something that our contemporary way of thinking and the resulting policies have been slow to acknowledge in earnest. In Native Hawaiian efforts to provide an alternative vision of health and a path for achieving that status they are issuing kāhea ola—a call to life and a challenge to the present.

Epilogue

It has been ten years since the original research was conducted, and indeed some things have changed and others have not. Native Hawaiians on island still have higher rates of obesity, cancer, asthma, and heart disease. Organizations that were around in the 1990s are still working hard to improve health access and knowledge. The program Hōʻea Ea has made numerous efforts at land-based health, including teaching people how to fish, farm, prepare food from the ʻāina, and work towards sustainability in these efforts across the islands. Numerous community organizations in Kalihi Valley have also joined in efforts to discuss the practice of land-based health. Not surprisingly, however, the use of Hawaiian values is still being used to sell the islands as a place to be consumed for leisure and relaxation. For example, lōkahi can be experienced in a moment of relaxation at the hotel spa and pool, bounded by the construction of an island paradise for a small fee at Hilton hotels. While the restoration of Hawaiian knowledge has moved forward, there are still sites of confounded meaning.

There have also been increasing efforts to improve the health of Native Hawaiians off-island: Pacific Islander Health Partnership and Weaving and Islander Network for Cancer Awareness, Training and Research are some of the health organizations in southern California. From sovereignty to food, there are increased efforts to get more information and resources to Native Hawaiians living off-island. In the 1990s, the sovereignty group Ka Lāhui Hawaiʻi had a booth at Hoʻolauleʻa to register Native Hawaiians for the Nation. For the past few years Kau Inoa, a sovereignty effort by the Office of Hawaiian Affairs that is supported by Hawaiian civics clubs on-island and on the continental United States, has been the primary group registering Native Hawaiians for participation in a Native Nation. And yet, when I recently pushed for the inclusion of conversations about the relationships between health and sovereignty at a research meeting for off-islanders, I was told by a researcher that we could not do that because it was not a part of the protocol and it would cause too many arguments that were not related to health. As the study progressed, many off-islanders brought up the topic themselves, calling for more critical thinking about the relationships between colonization, inequality, access, and health.

There are also increased efforts to make foods from the islands available in southern California. At the 2008 Hoʻolauleʻa I saw the typical plumeria and ti leaf plants for sale. This year, however, there were more pikake and even some kalo plants available for purchase. Interestingly, as I recently prepared for my Pacific course I wanted to have the students try some kalo and other "island" food. As I was telling my friend about my plans she told me that on Tuesdays the

Hawaiian/Japanese market, Marukai, received fresh shipments of poi, flown in straight from Hawai'i. But, she warned me, I should make sure to get there early because it goes really fast. So bright and early on Tuesday I arrived at the market. After walking around for a while I asked an employee if they had received there shipment of poi. He told me that their store was last on the delivery route. The Marukai store in Gardenia had received its shipment and had already sold all the poi. The Costa Mesa store expected its shipment at 4 P.M., but again, I was told to get there early because the poi sold out very quickly. Returning to the market at 3:30 I waited around, watching as more and more customers came to the market in anticipation of the shipment of poi. Finally at 4:30 the boxes came and we all lined up, approximately 12 people ready and eager to purchase fresh poi from Hawai'i. As we talked about how great it was to finally be able to buy fresh poi on the mainland, someone said that their relatives back home were not happy; because poi was being increasingly shipped to the mainland, there was less available on-island. While there are seasonal and even yearly drops in the availability of poi, the additional shipments to California were being blamed for the shortages, according to this individual's family member.

Why would they make more poi available off-island? There is certainly a market for the product. For example, a 16-ounce bag of poi on-island costs approximately $5, but off-island that very same bag can go for $17. Like the example of trying to obtain poi on-island that introduced this book, waiting in line for a food item that is a symbol of Hawaiian 'ohana and health and that is scarce again speaks to the political economy of health. The globalization of Hawaiian representations and practices refracts the problems of health inequalities. On the one hand, off-islanders can now participate in one of the primary symbols of Hawaiian health and identity. On the other hand, the extraction of this symbol of Hawaiianness from the islands exacerbates the already tenuous access to healthy practices. The counter-hegemonic push to implement Hawaiian practices of health through access to land has extended beyond the physical geography of the Islands. The question still remains as to whether or not portions of or all of the islands will be returned to a sovereign nation of Native Hawaiians and what the ongoing process of "freedom practices" will ultimately entail.

REFERENCES

'Aha Punana Leo, Inc. 1998. *The Story of the Punana Leo.* www.olelo.hawaii.edu (accessed December 1998).

Adelson, Naomi. 2000. *Being Alive Well: Health and the Politics of Cree Well-Being.* Toronto: University of Toronto Press.

Alu Like. 1985. *E Ola Mau Native Hawiian Health Needs Study.* Honolulu: Alu Like.

Aluli, Noa Emmett. 1991. Prevalence of Obesity in a Native Hawaiian Population. *American Journal of Clinical Nutrition.* 53:S1556–S1560.

Aluli, Noa Emmett and Davianna Pomaika'i McGregor. 1994. The Healing of Kaho'olawe. In *Hawai'i: Return to Nationhood.* Ulla Hasager and Jonathan Friedman eds. pp. 197–209. Copenhagen: International Work Group for Indigenous Affairs, Document no. 75.

Anderson, Benedict. 1991[1983]. *Imagined Communities: Reflections on the Origins and Spread of Nationalism.* London: Verso.

Anderson, Warwick. 2006. *Colonial Pathologies: American Tropical Medicine, Race, and Hygiene in the Philippines.* Durham, NC: Duke University Press.

Baer, Hans. 2008. *Killer Commodities: Public Health and the Corporate Production of Harm.* Lanham, MD: AltaMira Press.

Baer, Hans A., Merrill Singer, and Ida Susser. 2003. *Medical Anthropology and the World System,* 2nd ed. Westport, CT: Praeger.

Balibar, Etienne and Immanuel Wallerstein. 1991. *Race, Nation, Class: Ambiguous Identities.* London: Verso.

Balshem, Martha. 1993. *Cancer in the Community: Class and Medical Authority.* Washington, DC: Smithsonian Institute Press.

Barth, Fredrik. 1969. *Ethnic Groups and Boundaries: The Social Organization of Culture Difference.* Boston: Little, Brown and Company.

169

Basch, Linda G., Nina Glick Schiller, and Cristina Szanton Blanc. 1994. *Nations Unbound: Transnational Projects, Post-colonial Predicaments, and Deterritorialized Nation-States.* S.I.: Gordon and Breach.

Becker, Anne E. 1995. *Body, Self, and Society: The View from Fiji.* Philadelphia: University of Pennsylvania Press.

Beckwith, Martha. 1951. *The Kumulipo.* Chicago: University of Chicago Press.

Beckwith, Martha. 1970. *Hawaiian Mythology.* Honolulu: University of Hawai'i Press.

Bell, David and Gill Valentine. 1997. *Consuming Geographies: We are Where We Eat.* New York: Routledge.

Benson, Susan. 1997. The Body, Health and Eating Disorders. In *Identity and Difference: Culture, Media and Identitites*, ed. Katherine Woodard, pp. 121–181. Thousand Oaks: Sage Publications.

Bingham, Hiram. 1847. *A Residence of Twenty-one Years in the Sandwich Islands.* New York: Sherman Converse.

Blaisdell, Kekuni. 1989. Historical and Cultural Aspects of Native Hawaiian Health. In *The Health of Native Hawaiians*, Social Process in Hawai'i 32(1), ed. Eldon L. Wegner. Manoa, HI: University of Hawai'i Press.

Blaisdell, Kekuni. 1993. Historical and Philosophical Aspects of Lapa'au. In *He Alo A He Alo: Hawaiian Voices of Sovereignty*, ed. Roger MacPherson Furrer. Honolulu: American Friends Service Committee-Hawai'i.

Blaisdell, Kekuni and Noreen Mokuau. 1994. Kānaka Maoli, Indigenous Hawaiians. In *Hawai'i: Return to Nationhood*, eds. Ulla Hasager and Jonathan Friedman, pp. 49–67. Copenhagen: International Work Group for Indigenous Affairs no. 75.

Blaut, James Morris. 1993. *The Colonizer's Model of the World: Geographical Diffusionism and Eurocentric History.* New York: The Guilford Press.

Bordo, Susan. 1993. *Unbearable Weight: Feminism, Western Culture and the Body.* Berkeley: University of California Press.

Bourdieu, Pierre. 1984. *Distinction: A Social Critique of the Judgement of Taste.* Translated by Richard Nice. Cambridge, MA: Harvard University Press.

Briggs, Charles L. 1996. The Politics of Discursive Authority in Research on the "Invention of Tradition." *Cultural Anthropology* 11(4):435–469.

Briggs, Charles and Clara Mantini-Briggs. 2003. *Stories in the Time of Cholera: Racial Profiling During a Medical Nightmare.* Berkeley: University of California Press.

Brodwin, Paul. 1996. *Medicine and Morality in Haiti: The Contest for Healing Power.* Cambridge: Cambridge University Press.

Brown, Melissa J. 2004. *Is Taiwan Chinese? The Impact of Culture, Power, and Migration on Changing Identities.* Berkeley: University of California Press.

Brown, E. Richard, Shana Alex LaVarreda, Thomas Rice, Jennifer P. Kindeloe, and Meliss S. Gatchell. 2005. *The State of Health Insurance in California: Findings from the 2003 California Health Interview Survey.* Los Angeles: UCLA Center for Health Policy Research.

Browner, C.H. and H. Mabel Preloran. 2000. Interpreting Low-Income Latinas' Amniocentesis Refusals. *Hispanic Journal of Behavior Sciences* 22:346–368.

Buck, Elizabeth. 1993. *Paradise Remade: The Politics of Culture and History in Hawai'i.* Philadelphia: Temple University Press.

Burke, Marybeth. 1992. Hawaii's Health Care Plan Stirs Capitol Hill Debate over Access. *Hospitals* 66(8):32–36.

Bushnell, Oswald A. 1969. Hawaii's First Medical School. *Hawai'i Historical Review* 2(9) (Hawaiian Historical Society).

Bushnell, Oswald A. 1993. *The Gifts of Civilization: Germs and Genocide.* Honolulu: University of Hawai'i Press.

Canguilhem, Georges. 1991 [1966]. *The Normal and the Pathological.* New York: Zone Books.

Caputi, Jane. 1991. The Metaphors of Radiation: Or, Why a Beautiful Woman Is Like a Nuclear Power Plant. *Women's Studies International Forum* 14(5):423–442.

Cassidy, Claire. 1991. Good Body: When Big is Better. *Medical Anthropology* 13(3):181–213.

Castro, Arachu and Merrill Singer, eds. 2004. *Unhealthy Health Policy: A Critical Anthropological Examination.* Lanham: AltaMira Press.

Chavez, Leo R., F. Allan Hubbell, Juliet M. McMullin, Rebecca G. Martinez and Shiraz I. Mishra. 1995. Structure and Meaning in Models of Breast and Cervical Cancer Risk Factors: A Comparison of Perceptions among Latinas, Anglo Women and Physicians. *Medical Anthropology Quarterly* 9:40–74.

Chavez, Leo R. and Victor M. Torres. 1993. The Political Economy of Latino Health. In *Handbook of Hispanic Cultures in the United States,* eds. Nicolas Kanellos and Claudio Esteva-Fabregat, pp. 226–243. Huston: Arte Publico Press.

Chavez, Leo R., Juliet M. McMullin, F. Allan Hubbell, and S. Mishra. 2001. Beliefs Matter: Cultural Beliefs and the Use of Cervical Cancer Screening Tests. *American Anthropologist* 103(4):1114–1129.

Chrisman, Noel. 1977. The Health Seeking Process. *Culture, Medicine and Psychiatry* 1(4):351–378.

Chun, Malcolm Nāea (translator and editor). 1994. *Must We Wait in Despair? The 1867 Report of the 'Ahahui Lā'au Lapa'au of Wailuku, Maui on Native Hawaiian Health.* Honolulu: First People's Production.

Cleveland, Grover. 1893. President's Message Relating to the Hawaiian Islands, December 18, 1893. House Ex. Doc. No. 47, pp. 445–458.

Comaroff, Jean. 1985. *Body of Power, Spirit of Resistance: The Culture and History of a South African People*. Chicago: University of Chicago Press.

Comaroff, Jean. 1993. The Diseased Heart of Africa: Medicine, Colonization and the Black Body. In *Knowledge, Power and Practice: The Anthropology of Medicine and Everyday Life*, eds. Sirley Lindenbaum and Margaret Lock, pp. 305–329.

Comaroff, Jean. 2007. Beyond the Politics of Bare Life: AIDS and the Global Order. *Public Culture* 19(1):197–219.

Comaroff, John. 1987. Of Ethnicity and Totemism: Consciousness, Practice, and the Signs of Inequality. *Ethnos* 52: 301–323.

Crandon-Malamud, Libbet. 1991. *From the Fat of Our Souls: Social Change, Political Process, and Medical Pluralism in Bolivia*. Berkeley: University of California Press.

Crawford, Robert. 1984. A Cultural Account of "Health": Control, Release, and the Social Body. In *Issues in the Political Economy of Health Care*, ed. John B. McKinlay, pp. 60–103. New York: Tavistock Publications.

Crawford, Robert. 1994. The Boundaries of the Self and the Unhealthy Other: Reflections on Health, Culture and AIDS. *Social Science and Medicine* 38(10):1347–1365.

Curb, J.D., N.E. Alulu, J.A. Kautz, and H. Petrovitch, et al. 1991. Cardiovascular Risk Factor Levels in Ethnic Hawaiians. *American Journal of Public Health* 81(2):164–167.

Das, Veena. 1990. What Do We Mean by Health? In *Health Transition: The Cultural, Social, and Behavioural Determinants of Health*, eds. Caldwell, J., S. Findley, S. Caldwell, P. Santow, G. Cosford, W. Braid, and D. Broeres-Freeman, pp. 27–46. Australia: ANUTECH Pty. Ltd.

Desmond, Jane. 1999. *Staging Tourism: Bodies on Display from Waikiki to Sea World*. Chicago: University of Chicago Press.

DHHS, PHS, NIH, NCI, DCPC. 1992. Report of the Special Action Committee 1992: Program Initiatives Related to Minorities, the Underserved, and Persons Aged 65 and over. Bethesda, MD.

Dougherty, Michael. 1992. *To Steal A Kingdom: Probing Hawaiian History*. Waimanaolo, HI: Island Style Press.

Drewnowski, Adam and Specter S.E. 2004. Poverty and Obesity: The Role of Energy Density and Energy Costs. *American Journal of Clinical Nutrition* 79(1):6–16.

Drummond, Karen. 2007. *Learning to Care for the Dying: An Anthropological Examination of Palliative Care Education in American Biomedicine*. Ph.D. Dissertation in Anthropology, University of California, Irvine.

Farmer, Paul. 1999. *Infections and Inequalities: The Modern Plagues*. Berkeley: University of California Press.

Farmer, Paul. 2003. *Pathologies of Power: Health, Human Rights and the New War on the Poor*. Berkeley: University of California Press.

Finney, Ben. 1977. Voyaging Canoes and the Settlement of Polynesia. *Science* 196:1277–1285.

Finney, Ben. 1978. *Hokule'a the Way to Tahiti*. New York: Dodd, Mead.

Finney, Ben. 1979. Myth, Experiment and the Reinvention of Polynesian Voyaging. *American Anthropologist* 93:383–404.

Flegal, K.M., M.D. Carroll, C.L. Ogden, and C.I. Johnson. 2002. Prevalence and Trends in Obesity Among US Adults, 1999–2000. *JAMA*. 288:1723–7.

Flood, Josephine. 2006. *The Original Australians: Story of the Aboriginal People*. New South Wales: Allen & Unwin.

Friedman, Jonathan. 1994. *Cultural Identity and Global Process*. London: Sage Publications.

Friedman, Jonathan. 1997. Simplifying Complexity: Assimilating the Global in a Small Paradise. In *Sitting Culture: The Shifting Anthropological Object*, eds. Karen Fog Olwig and Kirsten Hastrup, pp. 268–291. New York: Routledge.

Frumkin, Howard. 2005. Health, Equity, and the Built Environment. *Environmental Health Perspectives* 113(5):A290.

Foucault, Michel. 1973. *The Birth of the Clinic: An Archaeology of Medical Perception*. New York: Tavistock Publications.

Foucault, Michel. 1977 [1995]. *Discipline and Punish: The Birth of the Prison*. New York: Vintage Books.

Foucault, Michel. 1979. *The History of Sexuality* vol. 1. New York: Vintage Books.

Foucault, Michel. 1988. Social Security. In *Michel Foucault: Politics, Philosophy, Culture*, ed. Lawrence D. Kritzman. London: Routledge.

Foucault, Michel. 2003. *"Society Must Be Defended": Lectures at the Collège de France, 1975–1976*, eds. M. Bertani and A. Fontana, general editor F. Ewald, translated by D. Macey. New York: Picador.

Fuchs, Lawrence H. 1961. *Hawai'i Pono. "Hawai'i the Excellent" An Ethnic and Political History*. Honolulu: Bess Press.

Gallimore, Roland, Joan Whitehorn Boggs, and Cathy Jordan. 1974. *Culture, Behavior, and Education: A Study of Hawaiian-Americans*. Beverly Hills: Sage Publications.

Galtung, Johan. 1969. Violence, Peace and Peace Research. *Journal of Peace Research* 6(3):167–191.

Garine, Igor de, and Nancy J. Pollock, eds. 1995. *Social Aspects of Obesity*. Luxembourg: Gordon and Breach.

Gilroy, Paul. 1990. Nationalism, History and Ethnic Absolutism. *History Workshop Journal* 30:114–119.

Gomes, L. Ku'umeaaloha. 1994. Mālama I Kekāhi I Kekāhi–Take Care of One, Take Care of All. In *Hawai'i: Return to Nationhood*, eds. Ulla Hasager and Jonathan Friedman, pp. 68–70. Copenhagen: International Work Group for Indigenous Affairs, Document No. 75.

Gordon-Larsen, Penny, Melissa Nelson, Phil Page, and Barry Popkin. 2006. Inequality in the Built Environment Underlies Key Health Disparities in Physical Activity and Obesity. *Pediatrics* 117(2):417–424.

Gupta, Akhil. 1992. The Song of the Nonaligned World: Transnational Identities and the Reinscription of Space in Late Capitalism. *Cultural Anthropology* 7(1):63–79.

Gupta, Akihil and James Ferguson. 1992. Beyond "Culture": Space, Identity, and the Politics of Difference. *Cultural Anthropology* 7(1):6–23.

Good, Byron J. 1994. *Medicine, Rationality, and Experience: An Anthropological Perspective*. Cambridge: Cambridge University Press.

Green, Karina Kahananui. 2002. Colonialism's Daughters: Eighteenth- and Nineteenth-Century. Western Perceptions of Hawaiian Women. In *Pacific Diaspora: Island Peoples in the United States and Across the Pacific*, eds. Paul Spickard, Joanne L. Rondilla, and Debbie Hippolite Wright, pp. 221–249. Honolulu: University of Hawai'i Press.

Halualani, Rona Tamiko. 2002. *In the Name of Hawaiians: Native Identities and Cultural Politics*. Minneapolis: University of Minnesota Press.

Hall, Stuart. 1994. Cultural Identity and Diaspora. In *Colonial Discourse & Postcolonial Theory: A Reader*, eds. Patrick Williams and Laura Chrisman, pp. 392–403, Harvester Wheatsheaf.

Hall, Stuart. 1996. The Question of Cultural Identity. In *Modernity: An Introduction to Modern Societies*, eds. Stuart Hall, David Held, Don Hubert, and Kenneth Thompson, pp. 595–629, Massachusetts: Wiley-Blackwell.

Handler, Richard. 1988. *Nationalism and the Politics of Culture in Quebec*. Wisconsin: University of Wisconsin Press.

Handy, E.S. Craighill, Mary Kawena Pukui and Katherine Livermore. 1934. *Outline of Hawaiian Physical Therapeutics*. Bishop Museum Bulletin 126. Honolulu: Bishop Museum Press.

Hasager, Ulla. 1994. Localizing the American Dream: Constructing Hawaiian Homelands. In *Sitting Culture: The Shifting Anthropological Object*, eds. Karen Fog Olwig and Kirsten Hastrup, pp. 165–192. New York: Routledge.

Hereniko, Vilsoni. 1994. Representations of Cultural Identities. In *Tides of History: The Pacific Islands in the Twentieth Century*, eds. K.R. Howe, Robert C. Kiste, and Brij V. Lal, pp. 406–434. Honolulu: University of Hawai'i Press.

Heurtin-Roberts, Suzanne. 2008. Self and Other in Cancer Health Disparities: Negotiating Power and Boundaries in U.S. Society. In *Confronting Cancer: Metaphors, Advocacy and Anthropology*, eds. Juliet McMullin and Diane Weiner, pp. 187–206. Santa Fe: School for Advanced Research.

Hobsbawm, Eric and Terence Ranger, eds. 1983. *The Invention of Tradition*. Cambridge: Cambridge University Press.

Holland, Dorothy. 1992. The Woman Who Climbed up the House: Some Limitations of Schema Theory. In *New Directions in Psychological Anthropology*, eds. Theodore Schwartz, Geoffrey M. White, and Catherine A. Lutz, pp. 68–81. Cambridge: Cambridge University Press.

Hoʻomalu, Mark Kealiʻi. 2003. Untitled chant. Track 13 on *Call It What You Like*. Honolulu: MKH Productions.

Howard, Allan. 1974. *Ain't No Big Thing: Coping Strategies in a Hawaiian-American Community*. Honolulu: University Press of Hawaiʻi.

Howard, Allan. 1990. Cultural Paradigms, History, and the Search for Identity in Oceania. In *Cultural Identity and Ethnicity in the Pacific*, eds. Jocelyn Linnekin and Lyn Poyer, pp. 259–280. Honolulu: University of Hawaiʻi Press.

Howe, K. R. 1996 [1988]. *Where the Waves Fall: A New South Sea Islands History From First Settlement to Colonial Rule*. Honolulu: University of Hawaiʻi Press.

Ito, Karen. 1985. Affective Bonds: Hawaiian Interrelationships of Self. In *Person, Self, and Experience*, eds. Geoffrey M. White and John Kirkpatrick, pp. 301–327. Berkeley: University of California Press.

Ito, Karen. 1987. Emotions, Proper Behavior (Hana Pono) and Hawaiian Concepts of Self, Person and Individual. In *Contemporary Issues in Mental Health Research in the Pacific Islands*, eds. Albert B. Robillard and Anthony J. Marsella. Honolulu: Social Science Research Institute.

Ito, Karen. 1999. *Lady Friends: Hawaiian Ways and the Ties that Define*. Ithaca: Cornell University Press.

Johnson, D., N. Oyama, and L. Marchand. 1998. Papa Ola Lokahi Hawaiian Health Update: Morality, Morbidity and Behavioral Risks. *Journal of Community Health and Clinical Medicine for the Pacific* 5:297–314.

Kaeppler, Adrienne L. 1993. *Hula Pahu: Haʻa and Hula Pahu—Sacred Movments Vol 1: Hawaiian Drum Dances*. Honolulu: University of Hawaiʻi Press.

Kahn, Miriam. 1986. *Always Hungry, Never Greedy: Food and the Expression of Gender in a Melanesian Society*. New York: Cambridge University Press.

Kamakau, Samuel M. 1964. *Ka Poʻe Kahiko, The People of Old*. Honolulu: Bishop Museum Press.

Kamakau, Samuel M. 1991. *Tales and Traditions of the People of Old. Nā Moʻolelo a ka Poʻe Kahiko*. Honolulu: Bishop Museum Press.

Kamakawiwoʻole, Israel. 1993. Hawaiʻi 78. *Facing Future*. Honolulu: Mountain Apple Company.

Kameʻeleihiwa, Lilikalā. 1992. *Native Land and Foreign Desires: Pehea Lā E Pono Ai?* Honolulu: Bishop Museum Press.

Kameʻeleihiwa, Lilikalā. 1994. Ua Mau Ke Ea o Ka ʻĀina I Ka Pono: The Concepts of Sovereignty and Religious Sanction of Correct Political Behavior. In *Hawaiʻi Return to Nationhood*, eds. Ulla Hasager and Jonathan Friedman, pp. 34–43. Copenhagen: International Work Group for Indigenous Affairs. Document No. 75.

Kanahele, George Huʻeu Sanford. 1986. *Ku Kanaka, Stand Tall. Hawaiʻi*: University of Hawaiʻi Press and Waiaha Foundation.

Kauanui, Kēhaulani J. 2000. *Rehabilitating the Native: Hawaiian Blood Quantum and the Politics of Race, Citizenship, and Entitlement*. Ph.D. Dissertation. University of California, Santa Cruz.

Kauanui, Kēhaulani J. 2002. The Politics of Blood and Sovereignty in Rice v. Cayetano. *Political and Legal Anthropology Review* 25:100–128.

Kauanui, Kēhaulani J. 2007. Diasporic Deracination and "Off-Island" Hawaiians. *The Contemporary Pacific* 19:137–160.

Kauanui, Kēhaulani J. 2008. *Hawaiian Blood: Colonialism and the Politics of Sovereignty and Indigeneity*. Durham, NC: Duke University Press.

Kearney, Michael. 1995. The Local and the Global: The Anthropology of Globalization and Transnationalism. *Annual Review of Anthropology* 24:547–665.

Keesing, Roger M. 1989. Creating the Past: Custom and Identity in the Contemporary Pacific. *Contemporary Pacific* 1:19–42.

Kelly, John. 1997. Tourism in Hawaiʻi. In *Hawaiʻi Return to Nationhood*, eds. Ulla Hasager and Jonathan Friedman, pp. 172–182. Copenhagen: International Work Group for Indigenous Affairs Document No. 75.

Kelman, S. 1975. The Social Nature of the Definition Problem in Health. *International Journal of Health Services* 5(4):625–642.

Kemeny, M.E., H. Weiner, S.W. Taylor, S. Chneider, B. Visscher, and L.L. Fahey. 1994. Repeated Bereavement, Depressed Mood, and Immune Parameters in HIV Seropositive and Seronegative Gay Men. *Health Psychology* 13:14–24.

Kent, Noel J. 1993. *Hawaiʻi: Islands Under the Influence*. Honolulu: University of Hawaiʻi Press.

King, Pauline. 1987. Structural Changes in Hawaiian History: Changes in the Mental Health of a People. In *Contemporary Issues in Mental Health Research in the Pacific Islands*, eds. Albert B. Robillard and Anthony J. Marsella, pp. 32–44. Honolulu: Social Science Research Institute.

Kirkby, Dianne. 1984. Colonial Policy and Native Depopulation in California and New South Wales 1770–1840. *Ethnohistory* 31(1):1–16.

Klein, Richard. 1996. *Eat Fat*. New York: Pantheon Press.

Koenig, Barbara A. 1988. The Technological Imperative in Medical Practice: The Social Creation of a "Routine" Treatment. In *Biomedicine Examined*, eds. Margaret M. Lock and Deborah Gordon. Boston: Kluwer Academic Publishers.

Kondo, Dorinne K. 1990. *Crafting Selves. Power, Gender and Discourses of Identity in a Japanese Workplace*. Chicago: University of Chicago Press.

Kua, Crystal. 1994. Hawaiians Describe Traditional Hunting, Gathering. *Tribune-Herald*, August 3, 1994.

Kulick, Don and Anne Meneley 2005. *Fat: The Anthropology of an Obsession*. New York: Penguin Group.

Kuykendall, Ralph. 1966. *The Hawaiian Kingdom 1854–1874*. Honolulu: University of Hawai'i Press.

LeBesco, Kathleen. 2004. *Revolting Bodies?: The Struggle to Redefine Fat Identity*. Amherst: University of Massachusetts Press.

Lee, Simon Craddock. 2008. Notes from White Flint: Identity, Ambiguity, and Disparities in Cancer. In *Confronting Cancer: Metaphors, Advocacy and Anthropology*, eds. Juliet McMullin and Diane Weiner, pp. 165–185, Santa Fe: School for Advanced Research.

Leichter, Howard M. 1997. Lifestyle Correctness and the New Secular Morality. In *Morality and Health: Interdisciplinary Perspectives*, eds. Allan M. Brandt and Paul Rozin, pp. 359–378. New York: Routledge.

Lewis, David. 1972. *We the Navigators*. Honolulu: University of Hawai'i Press.

Lili'uokalani Trust. 1962. *A Survey of the Socioeconomic Status of the Hawaiian People*. Honolulu: University of Hawai'i Press.

Linnekin, Jocelyn. 1983. Defining Tradition: Variations on the Hawaiian Identity. *American Ethnologist* 10:241–252.

Linnekin, Jocelyn. 1985. *Children of the Land: Exchange and Status in a Hawaiian Community*. New Brunswick: Rutgers University Press.

Linnekin, Jocelyn. 1992. On the Theory and Politics of Cultural Construction in the Pacific. *Oceania* 62:249–263.

Linnekin, Jocelyn and Lin Poyer eds. 1990. *Cultural Identity and Ethnicity in the Pacific*. Honolulu: University of Hawai'i Press.

Lock, Margaret. 1993. Cultivating the Body: Anthropology and Epistemologies of Bodily Practice and Knowledge. *Annual Review of Anthropology* 22:133–155.

Luomala, Katharine. 1989. Polynesian Religious Foundations of Hawaiian Concepts Regarding Wellness and Illness. In *Healing and Restoring: Health and Medicine in the World's Religious Traditions*, ed. Lawrence E. Sullivan. New York: Macmillan Press.

Lupton, Deborah. 1997. Foucault and the Medicalisation Critique. In *Foucault: Health and Medicine*, eds. A. Petersen and R. Bunton, pp. 94–112. New York: Routledge.

Lupton, Deborah. 1999. *Risk*. New York: Routledge.

Malo, David. 1951. *Hawaiian Antiquities*. Trans. Nathaniel Emerson. Bishop Museum Special Publication 2. Honolulu: Bishop Museum Press.

Malone, N.J. and C. Shoda-Sutherland. 2005. *Kau Li'ili'i: Characteristics of Native Hawaiians in Hawai'i and the Continental United States*. Honolulu: Kamehameah Schools–PASE 04–05:21.

Marshall, Wende Elizabeth. 2006. Remembering Hawaiian, Transforming Shame. *Anthropology and Humanism* 31(2):185–200.

Martin, Emily. 1992. *The Woman in the Body: A Cultural Analysis of Reproduction*. Boston MA: Beacon Press Books.

Martin, Emily. 1995. *Flexible Bodies: The Role of Immunity in American Culture from the Days of Polio to the Age of AIDS*. Boston: Beacon Press.

Maunier, Rene. 1949. *The Sociology of Colonies: An Introduction to the Study of Race Contact. Vol 2*. London: Routledge.

McGregor, Daviana Pomaika'i. 1989. *Kupa'a i ka 'Āina: Persistence on the Land*. Ph.D. dissertation in History. University of Hawai'i.

McMullin, Juliet M., Leo R. Chavez, and F. Allan Hubbell. 1996. Knowledge, Power and Experience: Variation in Physicians' Perceptions of Breast Cancer Risk Factors. *Medical Anthropology* 16:295–317.

McMullin, Juliet M. 2005. The Call to Life: Revitalizing a Healthy Hawaiian Identity. *Social Science and Medicine* 61:809–820.

Merry, Sally Engle. 1998. *Christian Conversion and Racial Labor Capacities: Constructing Racialized Identities in Hawai'i*. Prepared for the workshop on New World Orders? University of California, Irvine, January 17–18, 1998.

Morgan, Lynn M. 1987. Dependency Theory in the Political Economy of Health: An Anthropological Critique. *Medical Anthropology Quarterly* 1:131–153.

Morton Lee, Helen. 2003. Tongans Overseas: Between Two Shores. Honolulu: University of Hawai'i Press.

Morsy, Soheir. 1996. The Political Economy in Medical Anthropology. In *Medical Anthropology: Contemporary Theory and Method*, eds. C.F. Sargent and T.M. Johnson, pp. 21–38, New York: Praeger.

Nā Maka o ka 'Āina. 1989. *Pele's Appeal* DVD produced and directed by Nā Maka o ka 'Āina. Hawai'i: www.namaka.com

Nā Maka o ka 'Āina. 1993. *Act of War: The Overthrow of the Hawaiian Nation*. DVD produced and directed by Nā Maka o ka 'Āina. Hawai'i: www.namaka.com

NBC. 1998. The Next Wave. *Dateline NBC.* November 14, 1998. Lisa Aliferis (producer) and Laurence Solomon (editor).

Nelson, Diane. 1999. *A Finger in the Wound: Body Politics in Quincentennial Guatemala.* Berkeley: University of California Press.

Nichter, Mark. 1991. Hype and Weight. *Medical Anthropology* 13(3):249–284.

Nguyen, Vinh-Kim and Karine Peschard. 2003. Anthropology, Inequality, and Disease: A Review. *Annual Review of Anthropology* 32:447–474.

Office Technology Assessment. 1987. *Current Health Status and Population Projection of Native Hawaiians living in Hawai'i.* Staff Paper, Washington, DC.

Office of Hawaiian Affairs. 2006. Native Hawaiian Data Book. Honolulu: Office of Hawaiian Affairs, Planning and Research Office.

Office of Hawaiian Affairs. 2009. "Ceded Lands," www.oha.org (accessed April 2009).

Ong, Aihwa. 1987. *Spirits of Resistance and Capitalist Discipline: Factory Women in Malaysia.* Albany: State University of New York Press.

Osborne, T. 1997. Of Health and Statecraft. In *Foucault: Health and Medicine,* eds. Petersen, A and R. Bunton, pp. 173–188. New York: Routledge.

Perez-Stable, Eliseo J., Fabio Sabogal, Regina Otero-Sabogal, Robert A. Hiatl, and Stephen J. McPhee. 1992. Misconceptions about Cancer among Latinos and Anglos. *Journal of the American Medical Association* 268:3219–3223.

Pollock, Nancy J. 1995. Social Fattening Patterns in the Pacific. The Positive Side of Obesity. A Nauru Case Study. In *Social Aspects of Obesity,* eds. Ingor de Gaine and Nancy J. Pollock, pp. 87–106. London: Gordon and Breach.

Poyer, Lin. 1993. *Ngatik Massacre: History and Identity on a Micronesian Atoll.* Washington: Smithsonian Institution Press.

Pukui, Mary Kawena. 1983. *'Ōlelo No'eau: Hawaiian Proverbs and Poetical Sayings.* Honolulu: Bishop Museum Press.

Rouse, Roger. 1991. Mexican Migration and the Social Space of Postmodernism. *Diaspora* 1:8–23.

Rubel, Arthur J. and Michael R. Hass. 1992. Ethnomedicine. In *Medical Anthropology. Contemporary Theory and Method,* eds. Thomas M. Johnson and Carolyn F. Sargent. New York: Praeger Publishers.

Romney, A. Kimball, S. Weller, and W. Batchelder. 1986. Culture as Consensus: A Theory of Culture and Informant Accuracy. *American Anthropologist* 88:313–337.

Romney, A. Kimball, S. Weller, and W. Batchelder. 1987. Recent Applications of Cultural Consensus Theory. *American Behavioral Scientist* 31(2):163–177.

Rouse, Roger. 1991. Mexican Migration and the Social Space of Postmodernism. *Diaspora* 1:8–23.

Said, Edward. 1978. *Orientalism.* New York: Vintage Books.

Santiago-Irizarry, Vilma. 2001. *Medicalizing Ethnicity: The Construction of Latino Identity in a Psychiatric Setting.* Ithaca, NY: Cornell University Press.

Scheder, Jo C. 1993. Taro and Power. *Honolulu Daily,* August 1993.

Scheder, Jo C. 2006. Emotion, Grief, and Power: Reconsiderations of Hawaiian Health. In *Indigenous Peoples and Diabetes: Community Empowerment and Wellness,* eds. Mariana Leal Ferreira and Gretchen Chesley Lang. Durham, NC: Carolina Academic Press.

Scheper-Hughes, Nancy and Margaret Lock. 1987. The Mindful Body: A Prolegomemon to Future Work in Medical Anthropology. *Medical Anthropology Quarterly* 1:1–36.

Schmitt, Robert C. 1971. New Estimates of the Pre-Censal Population of Hawai'i. *Journal of the Polynesian Society* 80:240.

Scott, James C. 1985. *Weapons of the Weak: Everyday Forms of Peasant Resistance.* New Haven: Yale University Press.

Shintani, Terry T. et al. 1991. Obesity and Cardiovascular Risk Intervention through the Ad Libitum feeding of Traditional Hawaiian Diet. *American Journal of Clinical Nutrition* 53:1647S–1651S.

Shintani, Terry, Claire Hughes, and Wai'anae Coast Comprehensive Health Center. 1993. *The Wai'anae Book of Hawaiian Health: The Wai'anae Diet Program Manual.* Wai'anae, HI: Wai'anae Coast Comprehensive Health Center.

Shook, Victoria E. 1986. *Ho'oponopono: Contemporary uses of a Hawaiian Problem-Solving Process.* Honolulu: University of Hawai'i Press.

Silva, Noenoe K. 2004. *Aloha Betrayed: Native Hawaiian Resistance to American Colonialism.* Durham: Duke University Press.

Singer, Merrill. 1981. The Social Meaning of Medicine in a Sectarian Community. *Medical Anthropology* 5(2): 207–232.

Singer, Merrill. 2003. Critical Medical Anthropology. In *Encyclopedia of Medical Anthropology: Health and Illness in the World's Cultures,* eds. Carol R. Ember and Melvin Ember. New York: Kluwer Academic/Plenum Publishers.

Singer, Merrill. 2008. *Drugging the Poor: Legal and Illegal Drugs and Social Inequality.* Long Grove, IL: Waveland Press.

Singer, Merrill and Hans Baer. 2007. *Introducing Medical Anthropology.* Lanham, MD: AltaMira Press.

Singer, Merrill and Scott Clair. 2003. Syndemics and Public Health: Reconceptualizing Disease in Bio-Social Context. *Medical Anthropology Quarterly* 17(4):423–441.

Spickard, Paul. 2002. Pacific Diaspora? In *Pacific Diaspora: Island Peoples in the United States and Across the Pacific,* eds. Paul Spickard, Joanne L. Rondilla, and Debbie Hippolite Wright, pp. 1–27. Honolulu: University of Hawaiʻi Press.

Stannard, David E. 1989. *Before the Horror: The Population of Hawaiʻi on the Eve of Western Contact.* Social Science Research Institute: University of Hawaiʻi.

Steele, Claude. 1995. Stereotype Threat and the Intellectual Test Performance of African Americans. *Journal of Personality and Social Psychology* 69:797–811.

Stillman, Amy Kuʻuleialoha. 1998. *Sacred Hula: The Hula Alaʻapapa in Historical Perspective.* Bulletin in Anthropology 8. Honolulu: Bishop Museum Press.

Stillman, Amy Kuʻuleialoha. 2001. Re-membering the History of Hawaiian Hula. In *Cultural Memory: Reconfiguring History and Identity in the Postcolonial Pacific,* ed. Jeannette Marie Mageo, pp. 187–204. Honolulu: University of Hawaiʻi Press.

Stillman, Amy Kuʻuleialoha. 2002. Of the People Who Love the Land: Vernacular History in the Poetry of Modern Hawaiian Hula. *Amerasia* 28(3):85–108.

Tengan, Ty P. Kāwika. 2008. *Native Men Remade: Gender and Nation in Contemporary Hawaiʻi.* Durham, NC: Duke University Press.

Teaiwa, Teresia K. 1994. Bikinis and other s/pacific n/oceans. *Contemporary Pacific* 6:87–109.

Thomas, Nicholas. 1990. Sanitation and Seeing: The Creation of State Power in Early Colonial Fiji. *Comparative Studies in Society and History* 32(1):149–170.

Tom, Kiana and Jim Rosenthal. 1994. *Kianaʼs Body Sculpting.* New York: St. Martins Griffin.

Trask, Haunani-Kay. 1991. Natives and Anthropologists: The Colonial Struggle. *Contemporary Pacific* 3:111–117.

Trask, Haunani-Kay. 1993. *From a Native Daughter: Colonialism and Sovereignty in Hawaiʻi.* Monroe, Maine: Common Courage Press.

Trask, Haunani-Kay. 1994. Kūpaʻa ʻAina: Native Hawaiian Nationalism in Hawaiʻi. In *Hawaiʻi Return to Nationhood,* eds. Ulla Hasager and Jonathan Friedman, pp. 15–33. Copenhagen: International Work Group for Indigenous Affairs Document No. 75.

Trembly, Diane L. 1997. A Germʼs Journey to Isolated Islands. *International Journal of Osteoarcheology* 7:621–624.

Trouillot, Michel-Rolph. 2003. *Global Transformations: Anthropology and the Modern World.* New York: Palgrave MacMillan.

Turner, Bryan S. 1992. *Regulating Bodies: Essays in Medical Sociology.* New York: Routledge.

Turner, Bryan S. 1996. *The Body & Society,* 2nd ed. Thousand Oaks, CA: Sage Publications.

United Health Foundation. 2004. *America's Health: State Health Rankings. 2004 Edition.*

United States Census. 2003. Census of the Populations. Washington, DC: United States Department of Commerce, Economics and Statistics Administration.

United States Congress. 1988. *Native Hawaiian Health Care Act of 1988.* Congressional Record, October 30, 1988.

United States Congress. 1993. *Apology to Native Hawaiians by the United States Congress.* P.L. 103–150.

Waitzkin, Howard. 1983. The Second Sickness: Contradictions of Capitalist Health Care. New York: Free Press.

Walker, Isaiah Helekunihi. 2008. Hui Nalu, Beachbody, and the Surfing Boarderlands of Hawai'i. *The Contemporary Pacific* 20(1):89–113.

Wegner, Elden L. 1989. The Health of Native Hawaiians. In *Social Process in Hawai'i* 32. Honolulu: University of Hawai'i Press.

Weiner, Annette. 1988. *Trobriand Islanders of Papua New Guinea.* Fort Worth: Harcourt Brace.

Weller, Susan C. and A. Kimball Romney. 1988. *Systematic Data Collection.* Newbury Park, CA: Sage Publications.

Weller, Susan C. and A. Kimball Romney. 1990. *Metric Scaling: Correspondence Analysis.* Newbury Park, CA: Sage Publications.

Whorton, James C. 1988. Patient, Heal Thyself: Popular Health Reform Movements as Unorthodox Medicine. In *Other Healers: Unorthodox Medicine in America,* ed. Norman Gevitz, pp. 52–81. Baltimore, MD: John Hopkins University Press.

Wolf, Eric R. 1982. *Europe and the People without History.* Berkeley: University of California Press.

Worsely, P. 1982. Non-Western Medical Systems. *Annual Review of Anthropology* 11:315–348.

Young, Benjamin B.C. 1980. The Hawaiians. In *People and Cultures of Hawaii,* eds. John F. McDermott, Jr., Wen-Shing Tseng and Thomas W. Maretzki, pp. 5–24. Honolulu: University Press of Hawai'i.

INDEX

Page numbers with an f or t indicate an illustration or table respectively.

ABOUT THE AUTHOR

Juliet McMullin is an associate professor of anthropology at the University of California Riverside specializing in cultural and medical anthropology. The central focus of her work has been to understand the social organization and practice of medical knowledge as it is created and constrained within a political economy of health. Her research examines the contexts in which political struggles over health embody inequality, resistance and identity. These issues are explored through the topics of cancer, cultural meanings of health, and more recently, pediatric injury. The knowledge and practices associated with these topics reveal important processes that elaborate the links between inequality, access to healthy environments, and cultural constructions of risk and identity. The issue of cultural meanings of health and counter-hegemonic discourses are evident in her publications on Native Hawaiians and Pacific Islanders in the United States. Issues of cancer inequalities, particularly those inequities that affect Latinas in California are elaborated in her recent edited volume *Confronting Cancer: Metaphors, Advocacy and Anthropology* (School of Advanced Research 2008). Most recently Dr. McMullin was awarded a four year grant from the National Institutes of Health to bring issues of inequality and risk to bear on our understanding of pediatric injury.

Printed in the United States
by Baker & Taylor Publisher Services